Non-communicating Children

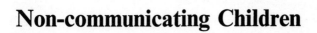

Non-communicating

Children

Louis Minski, M.D., F.R.C.P., D.P.M.

Honorary Consultant Psychiatrist, Royal National Throat, Nose and Ear Hospital, London

Margaret J. Shepperd, M.R.C.S., L.R.C.P., D.P.M.

Consultant Child Psychiatrist, Surrey County Council

NEW YORK
APPLETON-CENTURY-CROFTS
Division of Meredith Corporation

LONDON
BUTTERWORTHS

©
Butterworth & Co. (Publishers) Ltd.
1970

Suggested U.D.C. Number: 616·89—053·2

ISBN: 0 407 33200 6

*Printed in Great Britain at
the Pitman Press, Bath*

Contents

Contents

Preface

This work is based on an analysis of 474 children investigated in the children's units from their inception in 1953 until 1967.

The units, consisting of six beds at Belmont Hospital, Brighton Road, Sutton, were sited in a house detached from the hospital. They were opened on a research grant from the South West Metropolitan Regional Hospital Board when its Chairman was Mr. A. G. Linfield, who was very sympathetic to this work.

The work was initiated by Dr. Minski, as, in his capacity as consultant psychiatrist to the Royal National Throat, Nose and Ear Hospital, he was often asked by his colleagues to see young children to try and decide if they were mentally subnormal, congenitally deaf or had become deaf at a very early age. Diagnosis was often impossible and it often seemed likely that children who, in fact, were only deaf were being sent to institutions for subnormals. The units were therefore set up on a research grant for three years in order to try and assess these children and attempt at the same time to try and devise tests to aid diagnosis. After the units had been functioning for some time various types of children were referred for diagnosis among them being cases of children with communication difficulties resulting from a variety of reasons such as emotional disturbances, psychosis, aphasia, and so on.

The Nuffield Provincial Hospitals Trust generously bought a house in Sutton which they furnished and maintained for three years to which children who had passed through the units at Belmont Hospital could be sent. These children came from a disturbed home background and in this house they could have the affection and security of an ordinary household which they were lacking in their own homes. After three years the units became part of the National Health Service and still remain so.

The two units house twelve patients—the important point is that no uniforms whatever are allowed, there are no white coats and no hospital atmosphere. The day-to-day staff consists of children's supervisors who for the most part have nursery nursing certificates or have common sense in dealing with difficult and maladjusted children. Continuity of staff is as important as an atmosphere free from tension and friction. At the units at Belmont there is a night nurse but at the house in Sutton there is no night supervision—if a child is disturbed at night he is attended to by one of the supervisors. The technical staff consists of a part-time psychiatrist, a part-time psychologist, a full-time teacher of the deaf and a part-time teacher used to coping with maladjusted children. The services of a speech therapist are also at hand. The services of the EEG department and other medical services at Belmont Hospital are available to the units while Queen Mary's Hospital and the Hospital for Sick Children, Great Ormond Street have been most helpful in dealing with difficult paediatric problems, chromatography and lead investigations. In the units there is a permissive atmosphere tempered with discipline and training. Before any attempt is made to carry out any formal testing the children are allowed to settle down for some time and during this time they are observed, detailed notes are taken and it is hoped that they will, during the initial period of residence, begin to relate to other children and staff. Teaching is carried out on an individual basis at Belmont Hospital and when the children are transferred to the house in Sutton they should then be able to carry on in a classroom atmosphere.

As far as possible an attempt is also made to allow the children to lead a normal family life. They are taken out for walks in local parks, on shopping expeditions by the supervisors, given days at the seaside, and visits to zoos, while at Christmas a visit to the circus is made. There is a large garden at each unit with slides and swings and free play is encouraged while the psychologist holds play therapy groups as well.

Unfortunately, it is often necessary to retain the children for some months and, in a number of cases, a stay of years has been made. One reason is that it often takes a considerable period of time before an accurate assessment can be made and in other cases where a diagnosis has been made there is no suitable type of placement available for the child. If the patient is making satisfactory progress and the child is either returned home or incorrectly placed, regression may well occur and it is for this reason that the patient is retained until he is more stable or can be correctly placed.

The South West Metropolitan Regional Hospital Board also gave a research grant to enable Dr. Shepperd to analyse the records and it is on these results that the first eight chapters of this book have been written. Chapters 9–12 describe some of the investigations into the children's intelligence, hearing and learning difficulties and the attempts through teaching 'games' and operant conditioning being made to overcome these.

We are most grateful to our colleagues, Dr. Agatha H. Bowley, formerly Psychologist at the Belmont Hospital Children's Units; Miss Joan E. Taylor, Teacher-in-Charge of the Belmont Hospital Children's Units and Dr. Ian Evans, who have contributed these chapters.

Louis Minski
Margaret J. Shepperd

1—Introduction

A total of 474 children were investigated and these fell into the following categories.

	Male	Female	Total
Subnormal	107	50	157
Subnormal and deaf	46	19	65
Subnormal and marked emotional disturbance	17	7	24
Deaf	15	19	34
Emotionally disturbed and deaf	11	4	15
Emotionally disturbed	41	13	54
Aphasic	11	6	17
Brain damaged	16	3	19
Psychotic	55	11	66
Psychotic with brain damage	10	3	13
Psychotic with deafness	6	4	10
	335	139	474

SEX DISTRIBUTION

The proportion of males to females overall is 70 per cent of the total whereas in the psychotic group the proportion of males affected is 83 per cent. Again, in the emotionally

1

disturbed group almost 76 per cent were males but in the aphasic group, although the total number was small—19—the percentage of males affected was 84 per cent.

The only group, admittedly a small one—thirty-four—in which there was a slightly greater percentage of females (about 56 per cent) was the deaf group. However, where the patients were deaf and emotionally disturbed, again a small group—fifteen—the percentage of male patients affected was about 73 per cent.

It is well recognized that there is an excess of male handicapped children over females but so far no authority has been able to give a reasoned explanation for this proportion. We have attempted to analyse the aetiology—rhesus factors, rubella in pregnancy and toxaemia of pregnancy in the relevant groups with the following results.

AETIOLOGY

RHESUS FACTORS

Where rhesus factors were present 29 males were affected and 7 females. These were divided as follows.

	Male	Female	Total
Subnormal	17	3	20
Subnormal and deaf	10	2	12
Deaf and emotionally disturbed	1	1	2
Deaf and aphasic	1	—	1
Brain damaged	—	1	1

RUBELLA IN PREGNANCY

Where rubella was the aetiological factor 17 males were affected and 8 females. These were divided as follows.

	Male	Female	Total
Subnormal	7	6	13
Subnormal and deaf	7	2	9
Brain damaged	2	—	2
Brain damaged and psychotic	1	—	1

Toxaemia of Pregnancy

In the group when toxaemia of pregnancy was the causal factor 27 males were affected and 13 females as follows.

	Male	Female	Total
Subnormal	19	11	30
Subnormal and deaf	7	1	8
Aphasic	1	—	1
Aphasic and deaf	—	1	1

There is no correlation, therefore, between the aetiological factors in relation to the determination of the sex of the child affected.

2—Subnormal Group

The number of subnormal patients investigated was 246 and they were divided into the following groups.

	Male	Female	Total
Subnormal	107	50	157
Subnormal and deafness	15	4	19
Subnormal and marked emotional disturbance seen as outpatients	11	4	15
Subnormal and deafness admitted for further investigation	31	15	46
Subnormal and marked emotional disturbance admitted for further investigation	6	3	9
	170	76	246

It will be noticed that 69 per cent in the whole subnormal group was male.

DIFFICULTIES ENCOUNTERED

FAMILY STRESS

Perhaps the stresses to which the families of subnormal children are exposed should be mentioned here. The tensions within such a family are often marked and these may be due to differing opinions between the parents regarding the handling of the subnormal child. One parent may wish to send the child to an institution owing to its disruptive influence on the family; the other parent may wish to keep the child at home. Tizard and Grad (1961) stated that unless there were strong contra-indications 'parents should be encouraged and helped' to care for mentally handicapped babies themselves. A working party, convened by the National Society for Mentally Handicapped Children (1967), accepted these views. However, they were no doubt aware that beyond a certain point the burden of looking after a mentally handicapped child may threaten the well-being of the family. The working party also stated that for parents of older children the choice remained theirs.

Tension often occurs in the family as a result of the parents' over protecting the handicapped child to the detriment of the other children. In other families rejection of the handicapped child can occur which adds to its emotional difficulties. So often, therefore, it will be seen that the parents of a handicapped child require support and guidance, especially as it is so very common for them to feel guilty at having such a child and they tend to blame themselves as a result. Some parents may attempt to keep the child at home either by desire or by necessity because there are no vacancies in institutions or no training centre facilities. In these cases outpatient clinics should be available to which they can take their child and at the same time receive advice, superficial psychotherapy and support.

Day hospitals should be set up in addition to training centres. Here parents should be able to obtain some relief from the day-to-day burden of looking after a handicapped child. There should also be access to inpatient beds to which the child can be admitted when a crisis occurs or when the parents need a holiday and relief from looking after the child. The father and mother of one child in our series took it in turn to sit up with the child at night, acting as a night nurse. The other partner could then have a night's rest with one of their parents.

The report issued by the National Society for Mentally Handicapped Children (1967) points out that the examination by the school medical officer acting on behalf of the local education authority assesses children who may be subnormal at about the age of five. This is primarily administrative and is directed at excluding the child from school rather than at making a constructive educational or therapeutic recommendation. The report also emphasizes the inadequacy of a single assessment. The assessment of the child should be the task of a team of psychiatrists, psychologists, social workers, specialized teachers and the parents who should work in co-operation with the general practitioner. Greater co-operation is necessary between local authorities, hospital services and voluntary organizations. Suitable housing should be provided for families who have a handicapped child and are 'flat dwellers'. In these cases the children are more repressed and inhibited and emotional difficulties may well be increased. This, of course, adds to the burden. In addition, the number of short stay residential units, creches and day nurseries should be greatly increased.

DIFFICULTY IN PLACEMENT

A present difficulty is the cleavage between the Department of Health and the Department of Education and Science and the cleavage between these departments in the local authorities. If the Department of Health and the

6

Department of Education and Science would work more closely together and less in watertight compartments, the problems of the education of the handicapped child would be more easily overcome. Vacancies in E.S.N. schools are difficult to obtain, especially where the child is maladjusted. In addition, there are few (if any) local authority hostels to which subnormals can go. Many subnormals in institutions could go into hostels and in this way vacancies would be created for the more disturbed children who require institutional care.

Speech therapy is so often important for many of these children and this is extremely difficult to obtain adequately, if at all. Owing to the shortage of speech therapists a child may receive twenty minutes treatment a week which is absurd. While this shortage continues parents who are sufficiently intelligent could receive training in giving such treatment at home. This is done with the home training of the deaf.

SUBNORMAL OUTPATIENTS

HEREDITY AND ENVIRONMENTAL FACTORS

An analysis of the family histories of the above 157 children showed that 30 gave a history of dullness or subnormality. This was divided equally between both parents. Three mothers were dull and also tense and anxious while two were dull, epileptic. In 51 patients there was a neurotic heredity in that the parent was described as being tense, anxious, irritable and impatient. This tension was constitutional—it was not the result of having to cope with a difficult, subnormal child. Twelve parents were described as being over protective. Psychopathy and inadequacy were present in only a small number of cases. In seven cases only was there a history of florid psychosis, ranging from schizophrenia, paranoid states and manic-depressive illnesses (*see* Table 2 in Appendix).

PARENTAL AGES

Almost 50 per cent of the fathers were over 35 years of age when the child was born while 39 per cent of the mothers were over 35. The exact numbers can be broken down as follows. Seven mothers were actually in their forties when the child was born, while 29 were between the ages of 34 and 39. One father was in his fifties, 33 were between 35 and 51, while 19 were in their forties. Nineteen couples were over 36 at the child's birth and six couples were over forty.

Although it is well recognized that older mothers do tend to have more subnormal children, no weight has yet been placed on the relation of the father's age to abnormality.

AETIOLOGICAL FACTORS IN PREGNANCY

The aetiological factors were present as follows.

Toxaemia of pregnancy	26
Rhesus factors	17
Prolonged and difficult labour	16
Prematurity (ranging from 6/52 to 2/52)	13
Rubella	8
Antidepressive drugs	4
Anaemia in pregnancy	2
Injury to mother in pregnancy	2
Postmaturity (up to 2/52)	2
Tuberculosis	2
Glycosuria	2
Carcinoma in pregnancy	1
Severe influenza in pregnancy	1
Attempt to procure an abortion by unknown pills (*see* Table 5 in Appendix)	1

The effects of antidepressive drugs on the foetus are really as yet unknown but it is our practice never to prescribe such drugs to a pregnant woman. In several cases anticonvulsant drugs such as epanutin, mesantoin and phenobarbitone were taken throughout the pregnancy as the mother was epileptic.

8

Again, we are not aware of the effect of these on the foetus. One mother was ill for a time as a result of fly killer being used; at the same time other members of the family were affected. The nature of the drug could not be elicited.

Barber and Edwards (1967) investigated the birth records and school performances of 50,000 Birmingham children at the age of eleven. The verbal reasoning scores of single born children exposed to obstetric complications was compared with those of the population and their siblings. The results suggested that impaired performance was associated with only five of the obstetric complications studied—a short gestation period, a prolonged gestation period, toxaemia, occipito posterior presentation and delivery in an ambulance. In no case was the impairment very marked. However, children born at term did have a higher mean verbal performance score than those born after a shorter or more prolonged gestation period. Children from toxaemic pregnancies were found to be at great disadvantage when born at term. One interpretation may be that induction of labour in cases of toxaemia may curtail a period during which the foetus sustains cerebral damage.

It is obvious that much more research should be done on this aspect of the relationship of postmaturity, prematurity and toxaemia to subnormality.

Postnatal factors

Cyanosis	21
Jaundice (longest period 4/52)	20

Intercurrent illnesses

Meningitis	11
Measles encephalitis	8
Encephalitis	7
Lead poisoning	4
Vaccinal encephalitis	1
Cerebral thrombophlebitis	1
Phenylketonuria	1

SUBNORMAL GROUP

Other associated illnesses

Gastro-enteritis	6
Glandular fever	1
Muscular dystrophy	1
Acholuric jaundice	1

One child had suffered from carbon monoxide poisoning. In this case, the child was unwanted and the mother had attempted to gas him. This undoubtedly produced cerebral damage. Another child was suffering from mercurial nephrosis. This was the result of his having been given excessive doses of grey powder to allay his 'grizzling' because of teething difficulties.

PHENYLKETONURIA

One child was suffering from phenylketonuria. She was nine years old and it was impossible at that age to help her. Stephenson and McBean (1967) have emphasized the importance of carrying out the phenestex test in all children as a routine in view of the hereditary (recessive) aspect of the illness. In addition, routine dieting is only of value when started at an early age.

Hanley and colleagues (1968) in Toronto have stated that treatment of phenylketonuria with the standard low phenylalanine diet may produce profound malnutrition. This in turn may *cause* rather than prevent intellectual impairment. They suggest that a more liberal allowance of phenylalanine and protein, to ensure satisfactory growth and development, appears to result in improved functioning. They observed that patients who had been on the low phenylalanine diet therapy in the first few months of life had poor weight gain and linear growth and some showed evidence of serious malnutrition. In addition, ultimate I.Q.s were not as high as had been anticipated despite early diagnosis and seemingly adequate treatment.

When dietary therapy of phenylketonuria was introduced

10

ten years ago the aim was to maintain the fasting serum phenylalanine within a normal range of 1 to 3 mg/100 ml. Subsequently up to 6mg were allowed. But Hanley and his colleagues found that three out of nineteen children put on either regimen within the first six months of life had required hospitalization as they showed classical signs of malnutrition, deficient growth, hypoproteinaemia and anaemia. The other sixteen showed less severe but definite and prolonged evidence of malnutrition. Hanley modified the regime to allow fasting serum phenylalanine levels of between 5 and 15 mg/100 ml. Nine patients started on this diet within the first six months of life showed no chemical signs of malnutrition. On I.Q. testing, seven of the nine have been rated normal in intelligence, one dull normal and one borderline. The results, the authors say, are to be interpreted with caution. This is because the children are still under two years of age while three of the nine were considered to have only mild phenylketonuria.

LEAD POISONING

One of the male patients suffering from lead poisoning was aged five. His mother had suffered from toxaemia towards the end of the pregnancy. The patient was an only child who came from a happy home with normal parents. There were no feeding difficulties but he had been late in passing his milestones. Apart from bronchitis and rubella at one year his previous medical history was negative. The child had been suspected of being deaf at the age of two. After many examinations at a clinic it was felt that he was not deaf but avoiding sound—in any case it was impossible to get the child to wear a hearing aid. Chromatography was normal as were also tests for phenylketonuria. It was obvious that the child was 'disturbed' before the age at which he could put things in his mouth. It may well be that, as a result of the toxaemia of pregnancy, he was suffering from some degree of brain damage. He was seen by a child psychiatrist one year before he attended our units. At that time he had difficulty in relating, had stumpy hands, short fingers and dry hair. At times he breathed stertorously and his activities were almost completely aimless.

The patient was referred by the family doctor with an eight weeks' history of vomiting and more disturbed behaviour. His parents mentioned the possibility of lead poisoning as he had been eating the paint from the windows of the house. The blood lead was investigated and found to be 134 mg/100 ml. He was treated fairly continuously with penicillemine by mouth and in five months the blood lead had fallen to 70 mg/100 ml and later to 60 mg.

When he was seen by us he had no speech, was wet and dirty by day and night, slept well on his own but was faddy over food and a messy eater. He wandered around in an aimless manner, took no notice of auditory stimuli and it was impossible to gain his attention. He avoided visual stimuli also, walked around with almost a high stepping gait and with small steps. He showed no purposeful activity at all and still showed heavy breathing. He had no comprehension of speech, showed no gesture or miming and he was restless, overactive and showed marked pica. Formal psychological testing was impossible but he appeared to be functioning at about a two year old level. When last heard of he was attending a training centre with no improvement at all. Incidentally, a blood count showed him to have an HB of 77 per cent, no stippling of the red cells was seen, platelets were plentiful and there was slight anisocytosis. The total leucocytes were 10,000, 43 per cent being neutrophils, 43 per cent lymphocytes, 8 per cent eosinophils and 6 per cent monocytes.

Another case of lead poisoning was a male aged six who came from the West Indies, although the family was mainly of European origin. His progress and development in infancy were normal. At one year he was walking and at fifteen months he had a vocabulary of six words.

From the age of one year he had severe pica and ate anything including paint, toys, grass, stones and dead animals. From the age of 18 months he developed intermittent episodes of extreme irritability and screaming. Up to the age of two he seemed to be making progress with his speech and at two years he had a vocabulary of about 30 words. Over the next three years he lost his vocabulary and on admission had no speech at all. He was not toilet trained, was affectionate with his parents but did not make friends readily with other people. He showed a few mannerisms including repetitive movements and self-twirling. The family came to England primarily to seek advice regarding the child. The parents and two siblings were all healthy. There was no history of mental illness; the pregnancy, delivery and neonatal state had all been normal and his previous medical history was uneventful.

On examination the child had extensive pica, ate dead beetles, cockroaches, and was biting paint off the walls and toys. He had several attacks of vomiting lasting for some days and there was periodic abdominal pain. He was constipated and this was more marked when his mood changed and his behaviour became more disturbed. He soiled himself almost daily. His mood varied from moments of happiness when he liked being tickled and played with, to times when he was miserable, crying and whining. He showed tantrums when frustrated, threw himself on the floor and rushed away from loud noises. His moods changed rapidly from happiness to distress and again to happiness and these changes were considered to be due to colic. He now had no speech and communicated his needs by signals. He did not mix and showed mannerisms in that he rocked from side to side, banged his head with his fist and still showed self-twirling. He insisted on having a bottle until the age of five and was able to ride a bicycle well until this time. He was very dependent on his parents for every help—dressing, toileting and eating.

There were no abnormal signs in the central nervous system apart from some generalized hypotonia. The cardio vascular system was normal, peripheral pulses normal with B.P. 105/80. There was no hepatosplenomegaly. His blood lead was 168 mg/100 ml; H.B. 69 per cent with slight hypochromia and slight stippling of red cells. His white count was 10,000 with reticulocytes 5 per cent. Urine chromatography was normal while an x-ray of the left wrist showed dense lines on the metaphyses consistent with lead deposit. An EEG showed definite though moderate diffuse abnormality with a poverty of rhythmic activity.

He was treated with penicillamine mg 300 twice daily and pyridoxine mg 30 once daily. Psychological assessment was unsatisfactory owing to his non-co-operation and he appeared to be functioning at about a two year old level. Treatment was continued for two months and his blood lead dropped to 40 mg/100 ml but there was no improvement in his mental state. A further x-ray of the wrists showed that the line at the metaphyses had increased in density and width since the previous examination. The appearances were consistent with the diagnosis of heavy metal poisoning.

A further EEG showed the recording to be similar to the previous one. Treatment was continued with penicillamine and pyridoxine for a further two months but his blood lead remained at 40 mg/100 ml, his H.B. had improved and was 82 per cent while his white count was 5,300 with a normal differential. He had improved socially as a result of hospital routine, was more co-operative and took more interest in his environment.

He is still at home as his parents are able to look after him. His restlessness is being controlled by giving largactil mg 25 eight hourly.

INTERCURRENT ILLNESSES

All these children, of course, showed delay in passing their milestones except where an intercurrent illness, such

14

as meningitis or encephalitis, produced the brain damage at an age later than that at which the child normally sat up or walked. It is significant that 60 children suffered from measles. In many cases where the parents were able to describe the attack the child was often severely ill with a high temperature and drowsiness for several days. The probability in quite a number of cases was the onset of a measles encephalitis; in six cases this was definitely so as the illness was diagnosed in hospital. In 13 other cases the parents stated that the child's deterioration occurred after the attack of measles and there appeared to be no doubt that the brain damage and subnormality occurred as a result of measles encephalitis. For this reason it seems of the utmost importance that all parents should take advantage of the facilities to have their children immunized against this disease.

Lennette recently stated (1968) there was evidence that the measles virus could be linked with subacute sclerosing panencephalitis (S.S.P.E.). He stated that findings implicate measles in a possible 'slow virus' infection occurring 5–15 years after the patient's recovery from measles. Observations were independently made at Stanford Medical Center, Palo Alto, California and in Belfast, Ulster, in a series of ten patients. Microscopic fluorescent and serological studies disclosed markedly elevated measles antibody titres in the serum, measles viral antigen in brain tissue and viral particles in the brain 'virtually identical' with measles virus grown in cell cultures. The findings supported the work of other investigators who have suggested that S.S.P.E. may result from 'the emergence of a latent measles virus infection' in patients who had measles many years earlier.

S.S.P.E. is a relatively uncommon disease of children and adolescents that usually progresses to a state of functional decortication, coma and death within one to two years. The onset is usually insidious, marked by signs of intellectual deterioration, behavioural changes or visual disturbances.

15

In the Stanford series the patients aged 6–12 developed S.S.P.E. two to eight years after recovery from measles, while in the Belfast patients measles had occurred ten years earlier. Lennette states that it would seem reasonable to conclude that we are not dealing with infection with the common measles virus but with an altered course of infection not heretofore known to occur with this virus. It now appears that measles virus previously recognized only as an acute infective agent has the potential, under some set of altered host-virus relations, to take on some characteristics of the slow viruses giving rise to chronic neurological disease.

HEAD INJURIES

In sixteen cases, a history of head injury was given. Apart from one patient who suffered a fractured skull the injuries were all of a minor type—the child was not even unconscious.

It is obvious that head injuries play a very minor part in the aetiology of subnormality. The parents usually search for a peg on which to hang their hats as a cause for the subnormality and tend to exaggerate such a factor. In 39 cases there was a history of epileptic fits and in all except two the attacks were of the grand mal type.

Specific types of subnormality

Hydrocephaly	11
Microcephaly	11
Gargoylism	5
Mongolism	4
Oxycephaly	1

Physical deformities included spina bifida, congenital heart disease, cleft or high arched palate, cataracts, myopia and strabismus, dental abnormalities, such as lack of enamel or two rows of teeth, facial asymmetry and abnormalities of the fingers and toes, such as supernumerary digits, webbing or spatulate hands.

Neurological signs were common and included hypo- and hypertonia, ataxia, choreo athetosis, hemiplegia, quadruplegia, facial palsy and tremors of the hands. Mild emotional factors were present in 48 cases. These ranged from illegitimacy or total rejection by the parents to over protection or tensions in the home. These tensions were due to overcrowding or dissension as to how the child should be handled. Psychiatric facilities should be available to the parents and it is in this field that they are most required. Parents need help and sympathy regarding play, education and training in the social behaviour of the child. The family will also need help in relation to their attitude to other children, their own adjustment to the handicap and towards family planning. They will also have to be told tactfully and sympathetically about the outlook regarding the child's prognosis. In this way much can be done to relieve their feelings of guilt.

PSYCHOLOGICAL TESTING

The results were as follows.

I.Q. 80	4
I.Q. 70	11
I.Q. 60	22
I.Q. 50	17
I.Q. 40	19
I.Q. 30	10
I.Q. 20	4
Untestable	70
	157

It may be surprising to find 15 children with I.Q.s in the 70's and 80's who had little or no speech but in these cases there was a considerable emotional overlay and the lack of speech was due to these causes. Only twenty children had a

17

small vocabulary consisting of a few words such as 'mummy', 'daddy', and so on. The remaining cases had no speech at all or used an unintelligible jargon. If correct words were used these were applied in the wrong context and were meaningless.

It will be seen that the subnormal group is the largest group. While it was possible in most of these cases to come to an accurate assessment on an outpatient basis in 24 of the 157 cases, it was necessary to admit them for further assessment and observation. The usual reason for admission was that, although the child was often found to be functioning at a low intellectual level, there was a considerable degree of withdrawal. It was therefore necessary to establish whether the child was withdrawn because of the subnormality or whether the child was suffering primarily from psychosis super added to a degree of subnormality. It was obviously important to establish such a diagnosis as the disposal of the child was obviously different in the two cases.

SUBNORMAL AND EMOTIONAL DISTURBANCES

EMOTIONAL FACTORS

Although, as in the previous group, there was often a degree of emotional disturbance (usually due to rejection or over protection by the parents) in this group the emotional factors were prominent. There was a total of 15 patients of whom 11 were males and 4 were females.

Four children came from either broken homes or homes where there was considerable tension and quarrelling. The patients were tense, unhappy children and one was illegitimate. In one case where the parents were over protective, the child was over dependent and, if removed from the parents' presence, whimpered, screamed and then had temper tantrums. Another child was brought up by his grandmother who beat him and was cruel to him in general. As a result, he became cowed, anxious, tense and apprehensive. Other factors were overcrowding, favouritism, loneliness or admission to hospital for an intercurrent illness. In two cases there was a history of subnormality in the parents while in ten cases there was a neurotic heredity.

AETIOLOGICAL FACTORS

Among the prenatal factors one case showed rhesus factors while two gave a history of prolonged labour. The only significant history of illness in this group was measles in five cases, minor head injuries in two cases and one case of a tuberculous spine. One patient showed microcephaly and another showed hydrocephaly. Otherwise no definite syndromes were noted.

PARENTAL AGES

In six cases the age of the parents was over 36; the oldest was a father of 47 (with a mother of 38) and a mother of 43 (with a father of 38). The children in this group had higher I.Q.s on the whole than the uncomplicated subnormals. The lowest I.Q.s were 50 and 53 while the remainder were in the E.S.N. group (60–75). This shows that emotional difficulties can mask the intellectual capacity of the individual. Only three children in this group had no speech, the remainder had a few words or a fair vocabulary but indistinct speech.

PLACEMENT AND FOLLOW-UP

All these children were recommended for E.S.N. or private nursery schools. Where the home background was extremely bad residential accommodation was sought. It was only possible to follow up six of these children, five of whom were attending school and doing reasonably well.

SUBNORMALITY AND DEAFNESS—
OUTPATIENTS

Nineteen subnormal children who were also deaf were seen as outpatients, of whom 15 were male and 4 were female.

HEREDITY

Three patients showed evidence of subnormal heredity, five gave a neurotic heredity while in four cases there was a familial history of deafness. One of these was a case of Wardenburg's syndrome (*see* below).

AETIOLOGICAL FACTORS IN PREGNANCY AND PERINATALLY

The causal factors were chiefly as follows.

Toxaemia of pregnancy	4
Prematurity (from 3 to 6/52)	3
Neonatal jaundice	3
Neonatal cyanosis	3
Prolonged labour	2

Postnatal factors

Measles	6
Meningitis	1
Head injury (minor)	1
Lead poisoning	1

PHYSICAL FINDINGS

One patient was microcephalic, ataxic and had strabismus while one was hydrocephalic and had small, stubby fingers. In three cases there was a history of major epileptiform attacks. The only other physical deformity noted in this group was a congenital dislocation of the hip.

The family history of the patient suffering from Wardenburg's syndrome showed that a maternal grandmother was deaf and a maternal aunt and uncle had white streaks in the hair. The patient, who was severely deaf, had an I.Q. in the region of 30 and showed features suggestive of gargoylism with a curious configuration of the eyes. In addition, there was a left internal strabismus and there was a white streak in the hair. The condition has a recessive heredity and may show itself by a combination of deafness, subnormality and white streaks in the hair or by a mutation of these characteristics in the offspring.

PARENTAL AGES

Nine fathers were aged between 33 and 54; four mothers were aged 36 to 43. One father was 54 and the mother was aged 43 (*see* Table 4 in Appendix).

EMOTIONAL FACTORS

In eight patients emotional factors were present and consisted of anxious, over protective parents or illegitimacy. With one patient the child's difficulties were added to by the fact that only Italian was spoken in the home and the child was being brought up in an English speaking environment.

Psychological testing

I.Q. 70	2
I.Q. 60	5
I.Q. 50	4
I.Q. 30	4
Untestable	4

Twelve of these children had no speech at all while the two children whose I.Q.s were 70 were able to communicate by gesture and mime and by leading people by the hand when they tried to make their wishes known.

DEGREE OF DEAFNESS

Ten of these children were partially deaf. Two of them were thought to have a high tone deafness while six were

21

severely deaf. The causes of the deafness appear to be as follows.

Measles	5
Genetic	4
Neonatal jaundice	3
Toxaemic pregnancy	2
Neonatal cyanosis	1
Lead poisoning	1

In the remaining three cases there was no apparent cause for either the subnormality or deafness.

SUBNORMALITY AND DEAFNESS— INPATIENTS

The combination of subnormality and deafness made an accurate outpatient assessment impossible in many cases and for this reason 46 patients were admitted for further investigation. In this group 31 were male and 15 were female.

Heredity

Neurotic heredity	11
Familial history of deafness	7
Subnormal heredity on maternal side	6

Aetiological factors in pregnancy

Prematurity (from 3 to 10 weeks)	12
Rubella in pregnancy	6
Difficult and prolonged labour	5
Toxaemic pregnancy	3
Unsuccessful abortion attempt by doses of quinine	1

Neonatal factors

Neonatal cyanosis	8
Neonatal jaundice	7

22

Intercurrent illnesses

Measles	9
Meningitis	6
Encephalitis	3
Head injury	2
Gastro-enteritis	1
Pink disease	1

In one case the skull was fractured, in the other there was a history of blast injury in an air raid.

PHYSICAL FINDINGS

Seven patients gave a history of epileptic attacks of the grand mal type. Five patients showed microcephaly and among the physical concomitants were defective vision ptosis and ataxia affecting the finer movements of the hands. One patient showed oxycephaly and also suffered from congenital heart disease and strabismus. Other disabilities were asymmetry of the face and skull, athetosis and nystagmus, crooked teeth, habit spasms and ticks.

EMOTIONAL FACTORS

Emotional factors were present in 14 cases and consisted of illegitimacy, neglect and rejection by the parents, incest, tension and quarrelling in the home.

PARENTAL AGES

In six cases the fathers were aged between 35 and 50, while in five cases the mothers were aged between 34 and 44. In one case the father was 50 and the mother 39; in another case the father was 41 and the mother 44 (*see* Table 4 in Appendix).

Psychological testing

I.Q. 70	7
I.Q. 60	10
I.Q. 50	9
I.Q. 40	3
I.Q. 30	8
Untestable	9

DEGREES OF DEAFNESS AND SPEECH

Seventeen patients were partially deaf while 29 were severely deaf. Of all the 46 patients in this group none had any speech or at least any form of meaningful speech. Any speech present was a jargon. However, those in the higher levels of intelligence attempted to communicate by gesture and mime or by leading an individual by the hand to make known their desires. With those in the higher levels of intelligence frustration was very common and showed itself in temper tantrums and aggressive behaviour. Three children in the partially deaf group appeared to have a high tone deafness while one had a marked loss in the lower range of frequencies.

FOLLOW-UP

One boy whose handicap was the result of neonatal cyanosis and prematurity had fits, cataracts, congenital nystagmus, pes planus and valgus. He had an I.Q. of 60, was severely deaf and went to a school for children with multiple handicaps. He was supported by a good home background and is now aged 21. He lives in a hostel where he now makes simple, saleable handicrafts and has a certain amount of speech. This shows the value of a secure home. Four others with the higher I.Q.s were sent to E.S.N. deaf schools where they are making satisfactory progress.

LACK OF TREATMENT FACILITIES

Three of the children with I.Q.s of 70 were extremely disturbed emotionally and unfortunately the only placement possible was an institution for subnormals.

One of the most appalling gaps in treatment in the National Health Service is the fact that there are no facilities at the present time for treating the deaf subnormal child. It is time the Department of Health impressed upon regional boards the necessity of having in each region one or more wards set aside in subnormal institutions where deaf subnormal children can be centralized. They should then have the services of a teacher of the deaf either full-time or part-time depending on the numbers requiring treatment. In addition to this there should be welfare officers for the deaf who can communicate with the patients if their intelligence is sufficiently high to allow such communication. It is also time that teachers of the deaf put aside their objections to the deaf being taught to communicate by signing, gesturing and miming—we have found that many of these subnormal patients are unable to learn lip reading but are able to communicate by signing and so on. If these deaf children were taught in subnormal hospitals it is quite probable that their levels of intelligence would be raised. In this way they may be able to lead useful lives and learn to do some type of work in a sheltered environment, even if they are unable to take their full places in society.

SUBNORMALITY AND EMOTIONAL DISTURBANCE

There were nine patients in this group; six were males and three were females. They were all admitted for further investigation. In every case the home background was disturbed and the children were rejected by the parents, apart from three who were over protected by anxious mothers.

HEREDITY

Strangely the heredity of these patients showed no evidence of subnormality but in all nine cases there was a neurotic or psychopathic heredity.

	Mothers	Fathers
Anxiety states	3	—
Depressive illness	1	—
Psychopathy	2	3

The two mothers who had suffered from psychopathy were also prostitutes. One father was an alcoholic and two had served prison sentences (*see* Table 2 in Appendix).

PARENTAL AGES

Three fathers were 46, 39 and 38; two parents were both over 37. In one case the father and mother were 41 and 37 respectively while in another case the father was 47 and the mother 40.

AETIOLOGICAL FACTORS

Prenatal

Prematurity (2 to 4 weeks)	3
Toxaemia in pregnancy	2
Tuberculosis in pregnancy	1
Difficult and prolonged labour	1

Neonatal

Neonatal jaundice	3

Postnatal illnesses

Measles	3
Gastro-enteritis	1

TRAUMA

In two patients there was a history of injury—one child had suffered a severe electric shock as a result of sticking a metal instrument in a light plug. Three patients gave a history of epileptic fits of the grand mal type. One child was a mongol with athetoid movements and one was microcephalic.

PHYSICAL FINDINGS

Physical handicaps were not common in this group but ataxia, hare lip and cleft palate were seen.

Psychological testing

I.Q. 60	3
I.Q. 50	1
I.Q. 40	1
I.Q. 30	1
Untestable	3

EMOTIONAL DISTURBANCES

All the children in this group had no speech. In two cases the child had developed a few words but these were lost after a trauma, such as hospitalization for an operation or following complete rejection by the parents. In neither case did speech return. In one case the child became obsessional after hospitalization for an operation while the emotional disturbances showed themselves in temper tantrums, aggressive behaviour towards other people and destruction of their toys. Others were timid, cowed and apprehensive. One child was able to speak a few words normally at times and would then refuse to speak at all for months at a time, thus appearing to be showing the condition of elective mutism. Elective mutism is very rare; only four cases were discovered in a child guidance clinic with 2,000 children attending. When these four children did speak they showed no speech abnormality as this child did.

PROGNOSIS

The outlook with this group of children was hopeless as follow-up has shown that they are all in care either at training centres or institutions. Whether earlier referral of these children with the higher levels of intelligence would allow treatment to be more beneficial is, of course, a debatable point.

RESEARCH

It will be seen that in this mixed subnormal group of 246 patients the outlook is most depressing and fundamentally this is due to lack of money. There is not enough money allocated to research into subnormality as obviously we are still ignorant both from the genetic and biochemical aspects of the disease.

For instance it has been reported from the Arkansas Child Development Center that brain damage and learning disability may have an allergic basis in some cases. In this study of a pilot project of 20 children EEG findings became normal in several cases following anti-allergy treatment. All these children showed symptoms of allergy or a strong family history and 19 of the 20 showed abnormal EEG's. Four were of 'borderline' intelligence, four were on 'educable' level and two were 'trainable'. Seven had profound learning problems despite apparently normal intelligence. The various substances, such as milk, chocolate, maize, peanuts, and so on to which the children showed reactions were removed. After six months the EEG was found to be normal in nine patients and in two others the EEG improved. Eight showed no change and one was apparently more abnormal. Psychological test results showed no significant change. This is only one line of research which surely should be followed as, on the whole, our knowledge of the aetiology of subnormality is woefully lacking.

Although there is a certain amount of research going on in isolated units there is little overall research on a national basis. In our opinion this is due to the lack of opportunities for doctors who are 'research minded' and who wish to make their career in research rather than on the clinical side of medicine.

There ought to be the same ladder for research doctors to climb as that for clinicians, passing from the grade of houseman or registrar to that of consultant with the same rates of pay. If this were done the right type of man would be attracted to research instead of his being given grants from various bodies and then finding the money is insufficient to carry the research to a satisfactory conclusion.

Apart from the research aspect there is also lack of money being spent by regional boards on patients in subnormal institutions. These patients have the lowest maintenance rate per week of all patients in hospitals. In many cases the ratio of staff to patients is so small that they are even unable to be toilet trained. Perhaps it is looking for Utopia to suggest that children in the higher ranges of intelligence should have small wards and a reasonable ratio of staff to patients so that they can respond to mothering, security and social training. It was shown that subnormals do respond to these measures in the Brooklands experiment carried out some years ago by Tizard. The experiment is still being carried on in an 'experimental' ward at Queen Mary's Hospital for Children, Carshalton, by Tizard with smaller groups of children and a higher ratio of staff to patients.

Ultimately, it may be found that in this way money may be saved. Many children who respond could then be discharged to a sheltered environment, such as a local authority hostel and perform some repetitive or menial type of work which would help to make them partially or wholly self-supporting.

3—Deafness

Thirty-four children were seen as outpatients and were diagnosed as being deaf. These children were referred because of communication difficulties. Some were thought to be psychotic owing to their withdrawal and some were already at schools for the deaf but were making no progress.

Six children in this group were thought to be subnormal and ineducable by the referring authorities but, in fact, they were diagnosed as being deaf. Nineteen in this group were female and 15 were male, which is a reversal of the sex ratio found in children suffering from subnormality, psychosis, emotional disturbance, aphasia and brain damage. In this group there was evidence of hereditary deafness. In five cases the deafness manifested itself either in the parents or in other siblings.

AETIOLOGY

HEREDITY

In 17 cases there was a neurotic heredity. However, in half of the cases where anxiety and tension were marked in the parents the symptoms appeared to have been precipitated as a result of stress associated with the child's condition, although it must be assumed that the predisposition was already there. In five cases there was a history of intellectual dullness in the parents, but this did not amount to subnormality.

Prenatal factors

Prolonged and difficult labour	5
Prematurity ranging from 3 to 6 weeks	4
Rubella in pregnancy	2

Neonatal factors

Jaundice	4
Cyanosis	3

Postnatal illnesses

Measles	13
Meningitis	5
Otitis media	4
Catarrhal colds	3
Spinal meningitis	1
Fractured skull	1

PARENTAL AGE

The parental ages were not so significant in this group as in the subnormal group and were as follows: five fathers were between the ages of 34 to 43; two mothers were over 39; one father and mother were aged 43 and 39 respectively and, in one case, both parents were 39.

PHYSICAL FINDINGS

Physical concomitants were spinal quadruplegia in the child who suffered from spinal meningitis while facial asymmetry, strabismus, hemiplegia and ataxia were also found in some cases. Three children suffered from epileptic fits of the grand mal type.

In taking the histories of these children the parents often stated that following a cold or measles the child would hold its hands to its ears or would bang its head on the wall or bed. Apparently the child was suffering from otitis media which went undiagnosed. It must be emphasized that where a child behaves in this way otitis media should be suspected at once as immediate treatment could well prevent the onset of deafness in the patient. In 16 cases the deafness was severe while in 13 it was partial, five of these having a high tone deafness.

SPEECH

Twenty-eight children had no speech or only a few unintelligible words. In four children the speech was fairly good in that they had a few words and were able to communicate by speech in a limited way. One child had reasonably well developed speech and he was suffering from a high tone deafness which had been missed.

Psychological testing (performance tests)

I.Q. 138 (on W.I.S.C. performance test and I.Q. 106 on verbal tests)	1
I.Q. 120	3
I.Q. 110	6
I.Q. 100	6
I.Q. 90	8
I.Q. 80	5
I.Q. 70	2
Untestable (due to distractibility)	3

The child with the performance I.Q. of 138 shows the importance of using these tests and the complete uselessness of verbal tests on children who have any form of communication difficulties.

EMOTIONAL DISTURBANCES

Any child with either a physical or mental handicap (excluding severe subnormality) has feelings of inferiority.

They feel different from other children and are unable to enter into the active social life of normal children. The deaf child, who is unable to communicate normally but only by gesture or mime, is no exception.

Most of these children, therefore, were found to be shy and withdrawn. They became easily frustrated and threw temper tantrums when they could not make their wishes known. Screaming attacks, head beating and masturbation were not uncommon while teeth grinding, enuresis and aggressive behaviour were also found. The child's attitude to its deafness often depended on the home environment. Where the mother was over protective towards the child it became dependent upon her. As a result, it was timid, shy and often withdrawn and resented being separated from the parent. Again, in other cases, the child was rejected as the mother only had time for the normal children in the family. As a result, emotional difficulties occurred often in the form of aggressive behaviour, destructiveness, viciousness and spitefulness.

GENERAL MANAGEMENT

It would appear that many parents of deaf children require a good deal of help in coping with them so that they can adopt a line where discipline, encouragement and affection are reasonably blended. Six children were fitted with hearing aids and were then able to go to schools for the deaf or partially hearing units where they are now making quite good progress. Another child who had an antiquated hearing aid was fitted with an up-to-date hearing aid which made a great deal of difference to the amount of hearing which he had. It is important that hearing aids should be seen at fairly frequent intervals. Where children have aids which are not functioning properly, they will quickly reject them and throw them away. Great difficulty may then be encountered in getting the child to wear the aid again.

The Royal National Throat, Nose and Ear Hospital, Gray's Inn Road, London, W.C. has a hostel at Ealing, run in conjunction with its Nuffield Centre for Speech and Hearing, both of which were opened by the late Miss Whetnall. Here the mothers of the deaf children recently fitted with a hearing aid at the Centre can come for a week. The mothers are reassured and taught how the child can best cope with the aid. Any emotional difficulties are also dealt with by the hospital psychiatrist who visits regularly. This is an excellent scheme—it removes any teething difficulties in the use of the aid and also helps mother and child to overcome the emotional problems in the early stages of the deafness.

Unfortunately, at the present time the audiometric services under the National Health Service are sadly deficient owing to the lack of technicians. Another point which must be emphasized is that where a child has been given auditory training and lip reading for some time and is not making progress, signs and gestures should be used. It is of the utmost importance that the child should be able to communicate in some way, even with a limited number of people, so that its frustrations are overcome to some extent. We have found this of value where lip reading has been tried for years and has failed. (It is quite definite that some children will never learn to lip read, however long they are taught.) These children who fail to learn to lip read are usually those with concomitant brain damage and have language difficulties in any case. One child who had suffered a head injury had to be regarded as ineducable while in the other 33 cases recommendations for the children to go to varying types of schools (E.S.N. deaf schools, schools for maladjusted deaf, and nursery schools for the deaf) were made and the children are making satisfactory progress.

Henderson (1968) stated that a survey of older boys and girls in the schools for the deaf showed only 22 per cent had intelligible speech, 23 per cent had speech which was completely unintelligible and 55 per cent had speech that varied from barely to fairly intelligible. This shows that there is still a long way to go into the education of the deaf child.

DEAF AND EMOTIONALLY DISTURBED

Fifteen patients were admitted who were emotionally disturbed and deaf, of whom 11 were males and 4 were females. Ten had a neurotic heredity which showed depressive illnesses and anxiety states. Again, over protection was found in some cases while in others the children were rejected.

AETIOLOGICAL FACTORS

Prenatal causes

Prematurity ranging from 3–8 weeks	5
Toxaemia of pregnancy	1
Tuberculosis in the mother in pregnancy	1
Difficult and prolonged labour	1

Hereditary deafness

Hereditary deafness was present in only one case where there were six deaf mutes in three generations. However, the nature of the type of illness was not clear.

Neonatal causes

Jaundice	2
Cyanosis	1

Postnatal factors

Measles	4
Gastro-enteritis	1

Physical concomitants

Physical concomitants consisted of asymmetrical face, strabismus and defective vision, athetoid movements, ataxia, habit spasms and undescended testicles. One male child had a brother who was suffering from homocystinuria and the whole family was myopic. Seven patients were partially deaf and five were severely deaf. Seven of these patients had no speech and five had a few simple words but no sentences.

Psychological testing

I.Q. 128	1
I.Q. 110	2
I.Q. 100	6
I.Q. 80	6

The probability was that the six children who had I.Q.s of 80 were potentially of a higher level but their true level of intelligence was masked by their emotional difficulties. These showed themselves commonly in temper tantrums, aggressive behaviour, lack of concentration, and distractibility. In some cases there were obsessional features, posing, gesturing and exhibitionism.

PROGRESS

Six of these children went on to schools for the deaf and are making satisfactory progress while five had to be regarded as being ineducable due to their disruptive behaviour. Two other children were given trials at schools for the deaf but their behaviour was too disturbed for them to be retained and they were sent on to subnormal institutions. Two of these children have now left school and one is working as a gardener. The other is working as a kitchen porter and both are leading satisfactory and happy lives.

LACK OF PSYCHIATRIC FACILITIES

It must be emphasized here that there are no child guidance facilities available for deaf children with emotional difficulties. We would like to see one such unit established in each area where there is a social worker and psychiatrist who can communicate with the deaf and where the psychologist is familiar with testing non-communicating children. In this way, many deaf children with emotional difficulties might be saved and made into useful citizens, instead of being sentenced to spending their lives in subnormal institutions. Many of these children have reasonable levels of intelligence and early treatment, if available, may well save many of them.

PARENTAL AGE

The parental age was not so significant in this group but the age of five fathers ranged from 34 to 43 and two mothers were aged 39. In one case both parents were aged 39 and in another case the father was aged 43 and the mother 39 (*see* Table 4 in Appendix).

4—Emotionally Disturbed

Fifty-four children were investigated in this group, 50 of whom were seen as outpatients. Four were admitted for further investigation. Forty-one were male and 13 were female.

AETIOLOGY

HEREDITY

As was to be expected there was a marked hereditary history of instability.

	Mothers	*Fathers*
Tense, anxious, inadequate, obsessional and chronic worriers	21	13
Depressive illnesses	2	—
Agressive psychopaths	—	7
Chronic schizophrenic illness	2	—

Among both the parents, twelve were neurotic and anxious while three were dull. Of the mothers who were tense and chronic worriers, five were also withdrawn, introverted and showed lack of emotional warmth.

ENVIRONMENTAL FACTORS

Rejection by the mother was present in fourteen cases and in twelve of these cases the patient was sent to live with the grandparents. The result was that the child lived in an environment where he was either pampered, spoiled and indulged by the grandparents or he lived in an environment where he felt rejected, as the grandparents were too old to devote their time to young children and were irritable and impatient. A common cause of rejection by the mother was the fact that the child was unwanted or a child of the opposite sex had been desired. Three children were in care. In one case the father had died two weeks after the child's birth and the mother had of necessity to go to work—in the other two cases the children were illegitimate.

In fourteen cases the home background was unhappy and there was tension between the parents resulting in frequent quarrels. Four of the marriages had ended in divorce or separation. Other factors found in the home background were insecurity due to adoption, favouritism on the part of the parents, or jealousy of a younger child, probably caused because the parents did not prepare the older child for the arrival of a new baby.

Overcrowding or living in flats was an aggravating factor in several cases. Flat dwelling is, in fact, becoming a serious factor in causing emotional difficulties in children. Where the families live in a block of flats several storeys high it is impossible for the mother to accompany and leave the child in the garden (if one is available) at ground level. The result is that the child becomes frustrated as it cannot play in the flat. In addition, it is of necessity repressed by its parents as any excessive noise may be unacceptable to other tenants and neighbours. The only solution would be for supervision to be provided in gardens or playgrounds where the families are flat dwellers. In this way the child is less likely to become frustrated and disturbed. Again, it has been found that mothers living in high blocks of flats feel isolated and frustrated and their anxiety may be communicated to the children.

Adoption seems to present many emotional problems

for the child as even where the home is a good one, secure and free from tensions, children quite often seem to become disturbed. Obviously it is advisable for a child to be adopted as early as possible in its life. Many children, when told by their adoptive parents that they are adopted and were 'specially chosen', accept this and are quite happy with the situation. In fact, they may be quite happy about the situation until they get to school. Here they tell other children that they are adopted—the other children often ask the adopted children if they feel different from them as they do not have a proper mummy and daddy. The seeds of doubt and insecurity are now sown. The child often indulges in phantasy as to what his real parents were like. We have seen many disturbed children who become aggressive and hostile to their adoptive parents and unconsciously provoke them by rebellious behaviour, presumably as they are unconsciously seeking revenge for their being adopted. Adoption therefore presents many problems and in many cases the parents require a tremendous amount of support and help in dealing with the children.

Fostering, in theory, would seem an ideal solution for a child who is completely rejected. In practice, there are many difficulties in placing a disturbed child in a suitable foster home. Often foster parents, although warned about the child's emotional difficulties, are unable to cope. The child is once more rejected and this may occur on numerous occasions, thereby increasing the child's difficulties. It would appear that in some cases foster parents have emotional difficulties of which they themselves are not aware and are therefore unsuited to deal with disturbed children. In other cases, although they may appear to be quite normal individuals, they have no idea how to handle disturbed children. In our opinion some sort of training, both theoretical and practical, should be given to prospective foster parents and some sort of professional assessment of the parents should be obtained before they are allowed to act in this capacity. In some cases it may be wiser to place the child in a small children's home rather than place him with foster parents.

Hospitalization was a common cause of emotional upset in children. We have seen children who have lost their speech completely after hospitalization and also developed an attendant fear of doctors, nurses, uniforms or anything associated with hospitals. This raises the problem of admitting mothers to hospital when young children are inpatients. Firstly, there is the question of accommodation for mother and child which is sadly lacking and, secondly, if the mother is admitted, there is the question of someone to look after the remainder of the family who are at home.

PHYSICAL FACTORS

Physical aetiological factors were uncommon in this group.

Measles	11
Toxaemia of pregnancy	5
Neonatal cyanosis	4
Difficult labour	3
Glandular fever	1
Gastro-enteritis	1
Prematurity (3 weeks)	1

Two children were left handed, two suffered from a hare lip and cleft palate. Visual defects with strabismus were also present in two cases while one patient had a deformed kidney. Seven patients suffered from epileptic fits of the grand mal type.

GENERAL SYMTOMATOLOGY

Apart from the speech disturbances, which will be discussed shortly, concomitant emotional disturbances were marked and varied.

Temper tantrums, in which the child raged, screamed and banged its head, were common, while signs of anxiety and insecurity showed themselves in enuresis, encopresis, nail biting, nightmares, compulsive eating, food fads and thumb sucking. Two children suffered from infantile eczema while five had sucking difficulties in early life. Aggressive behaviour was common and showed itself in bullying or vicious and spiteful behaviour to other children and adults. In one case there was a history of arson. Some children were attention seeking, extremely demanding and histrionic. Others were timid, cowed and apprehensive and inclined to be withdrawn at times. Distractibility, restlessness, and over activity were also seen while lack of concentration was extremely common. Some children were neat, meticulous, and afraid of dirt and one child had a tic of the eyes with blinking.

SPEECH

Nineteen children had no speech at all and were unable to communicate in any way, either by mime or gesture. Fifteen had a few words, such as 'mummy', 'daddy', and 'bye-bye', but were unable to use any sentences at all. Seven children spoke in an unintelligible jargon and seven had fairly normal speech and had been referred primarily because of the concomitant emotional difficulties.

It was impossible to link any particular type of speech defect with any specific emotional difficulties, nor was the degree or type of speech defect associated with any particular level of intelligence. Psychological testing showed the following level of intelligence.

I.Q. 140	1
I.Q. 130	2
I.Q. 120	5
I.Q. 110	9
I.Q. 100	17
I.Q. 90	7
I.Q. 80	4
I.Q. 70	4
Untestable	5

It was significant that the child with the I.Q. of 140 had no speech at all, the two children with I.Q.s of 130 had only a few words while three of the children with I.Q.s of 120 had only jargon type of speech. Seven of the children with I.Q.s of 100 had only a few simple words as did three of the children with I.Q.s of 80. It is obvious, therefore, that there is no correlation between the level of intelligence and the amount of speech the child had. This obviously depends much more on the degree of emotional disturbance. What is much more significant is the fact that after a specific emotional trauma, such as hospitalization or separation from the parents, any speech which the child had had tended to disappear completely.

RECOMMENDATIONS

Ten of the parents refused to accept advice given to them regarding treatment and placement of the child. This is not unexpected when one is dealing with a difficult and disturbed home background. The recommendations were as follows.

Fourteen children were referred to nursery schools or nursery classes while 21 were referred to child guidance clinics. Fifteen children were referred to nursery schools and speech therapy was recommended at the same time. One child was sent to an adolescent unit, two were referred to E.S.N. schools with a recommendation for speech therapy and another child was referred to a remedial class with the advice that speech therapy should be given. Sixteen parents ignored our follow-up letters but seventeen children are reported to be doing well with marked improvement in their speech. At the present time the remaining children are unchanged. However, it must be remembered that ten parents refused to follow our advice and sixteen were unable to be assessed because of lack of follow-up information.

In referring children to child guidance clinics it should be stressed that there is often a long waiting list before a child can be seen. In one clinic, there was a wait of two years and this was with the case of a child with a school phobia. In addition, when the child is seen after the initial interview, it is often not seen again for a month and the amount of treatment given is negligible. In view of the shortage of child psychiatrists and ancillary staff, such as social workers, and psychologists, many of these children and parents should be seen at day hospitals. They could attend these two or three times a week and the children and parents could be treated more efficiently, possibly in groups. In addition, when a disturbed child requires inpatient accommodation, the facilities for inpatient treatment of such children is sadly lacking and more beds should be provided.

Again on the educational side it is often difficult to obtain vacancies in nursery or remedial classes. It is a disgraceful state of affairs where a young child has to wait a year or more before it can receive education or treatment. In our view these children require 'therapeutic education' and if education and health both at a national and local authority level were not in such watertight compartments, much might be done to streamline the services for these children.

5—Aphasia

Seventeen children were seen who were suffering from aphasia of whom eleven were male and six were female.

AETIOLOGY

Heredity

	Mothers	Fathers
Depressive illnesses	4	—
Subnormality	2	—
Withdrawn and schizophrenic	1	1

Of the four mothers who suffered from depressive illnesses, it was not known whether anti-depressive drugs had been taken. For the parental ages, *see* Table 4 in Appendix.

EMOTIONAL FACTORS

One child was over protected by the parents, two were rejected, one was illegitimate; in four cases the family background was disturbed and there was tension and quarrelling in the home. Emotional disturbances are not uncommon in aphasic children due often to their frustration at being unable to communicate and where the family background is disturbed these may well be exaggerated.

Prenatal factors

Prematurity ranging from 3–10 weeks	4
Toxaemia of pregnancy	4
Rubella in pregnancy	1
Antepartum haemorrhage	1

It should be noted that prematurity is often associated with toxaemia as labour is often induced early to save the mother's life.

Neonatal factors

Jaundice	5
Cyanosis	3

Two of the cases of neonatal jaundice had exchange transfusions at birth.

Postnatal factors

Measles	6
Otitis media	2
Meningitis	2
Pyloric stenosis	1

Two children gave a history of epileptic fits of the grand mal type. Seven children suffered from concomitant deafness and, in most cases, the diagnosis of the deafness was extremely difficult.

CASE HISTORY—APHASIA AND DEAFNESS

One girl with an I.Q. of 107 was in our units for several months. Although it was thought that she was probably deaf as well as aphasic it was impossible to make a definite diagnosis. This child had many emotional difficulties—the mother had suffered from a depressive illness and the child had been rejected by her parents. She was sent to Edith Edwards House School in Banstead and, after being there for many months, she became more settled. Previously, she had been withdrawn, shy, timid and aggressive by turn and also showed many mannerisms and obsessional traits. Eventually an audiogram was obtained and this showed a severe hearing loss. She was fitted with hearing aids and when the child was able to hear the change was dramatic. She became much less withdrawn, mixed more readily and showed pleasurable reaction and eventually began to develop speech. She is now in a partially hearing school and making excellent progress. This child had an abnormal EEG (result of toxaemia in pregnancy) and K complexes were present. This did not help, however, as the defect was central in origin and deafness could therefore not be ruled out. The diagnosis of deafness in aphasic children is extremely difficult and it may take months of laborious testing before a diagnosis is confirmed.

TYPES OF APHASIA

Four children had good comprehension of speech and their disability was on the expressive side. Where there was little or no comprehension of speech, the children used miming and gesturing and led people by the hand to make known their wishes. None of the children in this group had any speech and apart from the children with good comprehension, their disability was a dual one in that they had difficulties on both receptive and expressive sides of speech. Tantrums were very common and were usually the result of frustration at being unable to make themselves understood.

CASE HISTORY—EXPRESSIVE APHASIA WITH EMOTIONAL OVERLAY

One boy who had normal speech comprehension from infancy and whose executive speech was confined to six dyslalic words also showed idioglossia.

His mother was a gentle, over permissive, and over protective person while the father was a serious, mildly obsessional, man. The child showed a clinging dependency to his mother, a separation anxiety, and, at times, had tantrums when frustrated. He also became withdrawn and negativistic and at nights his sleep was disturbed and he cried for his mother. He also showed obsessional behaviour in that he would carry objects around and showed food obsessions and would become very miserable and upset when thwarted. He withdrew rapidly into non-effort and manipulated the environment to his advantage. This child improved considerably and arrangements were made for him to go to Edith Edwards House School.

PHYSICAL CONCOMITANTS

Neurological signs were not common although clumsiness and athetoid movements were present in three cases—one had a strabismus and one facial asymmetry. In one case where the aetiology was not clear but was probably rubella in pregnancy, the child was partially deaf and had a cleft palate. In addition to this he was left handed and showed mirror writing. Three children had large heads but could not be classified as hydrocephalics. All these children showed the distractibility, hyperkinesis and over activity of the brain damaged child.

SECONDARY PSYCHOTIC FEATURES

A number of these children were referred because they were thought to be psychotic as they appeared to be withdrawn and had difficulty in making relationships with other people. It is not uncommon to see withdrawal with aphasic children. This is a secondary symptom, due to the children's inability to communicate, which disappears fairly rapidly when the child begins to communicate.

Psychological testing

I.Q. 140	1
I.Q. 120	2
I.Q. 110	2
I.Q. 100	7
I.Q. 90	3
I.Q. 80	2

CASE HISTORY

The child with the I.Q. of 140 was the daughter of professional parents. The mother suffered from toxaemia in pregnancy and the child was also six weeks premature. The home atmosphere was explosive; the father was aged 41 and both parents were tense and anxious. The child was also tense and anxious and showed many obsessional traits. She had a fair comprehension of speech and was sent to a class for aphasic children where she is now doing well.

Placement

All these children were sent to special schools, such as Moor House, Oxted, or John Horniman, Worthing, or to special classes for aphasic children where they are making satisfactory progress. One of the present difficulties is that there are too few classes or schools for this type of child and as a result the waiting lists are extremely long.

6—Brain Damage

Although many of the subnormal and deaf patients showed brain damage (as, of course, did those suffering from aphasia) 19 patients were placed into this category—16 were males and 3 were females.

AETIOLOGY

GENERAL CHARACTERISTICS
The patients in this group were all of reasonable intelligence but they all showed the hyperkinesis, over activity and distractibility of the brain damaged child. Spatial difficulties were also marked while in some cases neurological signs were present. In fifteen cases the EEG's were abnormal and in four cases there was a focal abnormality in the left Sylvian area, left posterior temporal region and two in the right mid-temporal region. The remainder showed a diffuse generalized abnormality with spike and wave activity where fits were present. These, in fact, occurred in only two cases and were of the grand mal type.

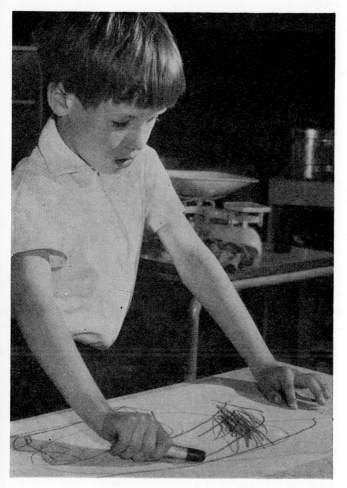

Figure 1. Brain damaged child.

HEREDITY

Surprisingly enough in this group there was a high incidence of neurotic heredity.

	Mothers	Fathers
Neurosis	6	2
Schizophrenia	1	1

In three cases both parents were anxious and over protective; in three cases both parents were dull. One schizophrenic mother had been on phenothiazines during pregnancy.

Where the parents were anxious and over protective it was difficult to decide if their anxiety existed before the child's handicap was diagnosed or whether the anxiety occurred as a direct result of the diagnosis.

PARENTAL AGE

In six cases the fathers' ages were 46, 45, 42 (2), 38 and 37 and the father of 46 was married to a mother of 40.

Prenatal factors

Toxaemia of pregnancy	6
Difficult and prolonged labour	5
Rubella in pregnancy	2
Prematurity (7 weeks)	2

Neonatal factors

Cyanosis	6
Jaundice	1

Obviously, in some cases there was a combination of factors such as toxaemia and difficult labour; another suffered from prolonged labour and cyanosis; another a combination of rubella and cyanosis and one suffered from toxaemia prematurity and postnatal cyanosis. Eight children gave a history of measles but in only one case did the illness appear to be severe and suggestive of encephalitis.

POSSIBLE AETIOLOGICAL FACTORS

One mother developed diabetes during the pregnancy and another suffered from a transient glycosuris. Whether these conditions produce brain damage in the foetus is not known at the present time. One mother had had pneumonia during the pregnancy and had been treated with antibiotics. The child was born with a hemiplegia and developed epileptic fits. It might be suggested that the foetus developed a pneumococcal meningitis *in utero* but this, of course, is highly speculative. Again, the effects of antibiotics on the foetus are not really known. Another mother had severe influenza during the pregnancy, one had gonorrhoea, and another had taken pills of some nature to procure an abortion.

At the present time we appear to be ignorant as to the part played by various illnesses and drugs in damaging the foetus. When one considers that cerebral anoxia of a very short duration can produce brain damage, more research is necessary into its aetiology. It has been shown that where children are suffering from erythroblastosis foetalis immediate exchange transfusions do not always obviate brain damage in the child. Where it is suffering from neonatal cyanosis and is put in an oxygen tent or given mouth to mouth resuscitation, brain damage can still occur.

Eleven children had no speech or only an unintelligible jargon. Seven had a few simple words or indistinct speech which was intelligible to parents or those who were in contact with them for some time. In one case the speech was reasonably good and the child was able to use sentences. One child, who suffered from brain damage as a result of rubella and cyanosis, was developing speech quite well but at the age of three he fell into a reservoir. After this his speech completely disappeared and he became very withdrawn.

Physical concomitants

Nine children showed neurological manifestations. These included clumsiness in carrying out fine movements, choreiform and athetoid movements, and hypertonia. Paraplegia with slow tongue movements was present in one case while four cases had strabismus. Other physical concomitants were batlike ears, asymmetry of the face and flattened occiput, congenital cataract, webbed toes and congenital heart disease (patent ductus arteriosus). Only two gave a history of epileptic fits.

Psychological testing

I.Q. 138	1
I.Q. 135	1
I.Q. 120	4
I.Q. 110	1
I.Q. 100	3
I.Q. 90	6
I.Q. 80	3

Emotional disturbances and placement

In two cases obsessional tidiness in play was noticed and in both cases the parents had marked obsessional traits in their personality. Two other children were withdrawn, did not mix with the other children but played on their own. In these cases the fathers were withdrawn, reserved and introverted.

Grimacing was extremely common and the children were demanding, attention seeking and became frustrated and showed tantrums if thwarted. The child with the I.Q. of 138 went to a school with a small remedial class and was given speech therapy. This child is improving. The child with the I.Q. of 135 had normal speech, and was referred primarily because of behaviour problems. These were due to his difficult home background and he was referred to a child guidance clinic. In seven cases there were marked emotional difficulties superadded to the brain damage. The parents of one child with an I.Q. of 119 refused to take our advice as to placement and wished to send the child to an ordinary primary school, presumably to convince themselves and other people that the child was normal. The child with an I.Q. of 120 was the child who fell into the reservoir. He went to a school for physically handicapped children and is doing well. The remaining children were also eventually sent to schools with small remedial classes with a recommendation to have speech therapy. Those we were able to follow up are making satisfactory progress.

An attempt was made to correlate the position of the brain damaged child in the family but it was impossible to do this as there was so much variation. In some of the cases where toxaemia of pregnancy was the causal factor in this and other groups such as the subnormal, pills had been given to the mother as part of her treatment. The nature of these pills was not known.

7—Psychotic Children

We prefer to use the name psychotic children or psychosis of childhood, as autism is simply a symptom of the illness. It has been suggested that psychosis of childhood would then include other conditions, such as depressive states. However, it is most unusual to find a psychotic depression in childhood and any depressive features present are usually in the setting of a severe emotional disturbance. Again, schizophrenia in childhood is rare and, if seen, is a completely different entity and cannot be confused with 'autistic' children. The children described in this chapter of the book are therefore synonymous with those described by some writers as 'autistic' children.

Undoubtedly, the illness has occurred over a long period of time and it may well be that some of the children classed as idiot savants belonged to this group. Obviously, many of these unrecognized children were regarded as being subnormal and were relegated to subnormal institutions. Kanner was the individual who first described the syndrome of infantile autism, which was then referred to as Kanner's Syndrome.

TYPES OF PSYCHOTIC CHILDREN

There were 89 children in this group subdivided as follows.

	Male	Female	Total
With no evidence of brain damage	55	11	66
With brain damage	10	3	13
With deafness	6	4	10
	—	—	—
	71	18	89

A total of 89 psychotic children was investigated and the proportion of males to females is almost four to one. This proportion is similar to those of other observers. Creak and Ini (1960) found 3·6 boys to 1 girl in a series of 121 children and Annell (1963) found 4·5 to 1 girl in 115 children. No apparent explanation is possible at the present time.

In the 66 cases without brain damage, in 24 the age of the father was 35 or upwards, the highest age being 52, while in 18 cases the age of the mother was over 35, the highest age being 46.

In 15 cases the age of both parents was over 35 and in three cases the age of both parents was over 40 (*see* Table 4 in Appendix). It may be that apart from hereditary or environmental factors older parents are less tolerant towards young children, become impatient more readily, and show less emotional warmth towards them.

The position of the child in the family did not appear to bear any relationship to the illness as eight were only children and three were illegitimate. With the remainder the position varied considerably as did the size of the family and the number of males and females. Nine patients were the middle child in a family of three children while in the remainder the patient varied from being the fifth of six to the elder of two, the eldest of three or the second of four. Rimland (1964) stated that childhood autism appeared to be commoner among the first born but this certainly is not the case in our series.

In 45 out of the 66 cases (just over 68 per cent) there was some form of psychiatric disturbance in the parents. In 32 cases this was evident in both parents while in seven cases the mother was the unstable parent and in eight cases the father was the disturbed partner.

The following shows the type of psychiatric symptoms present.

Both parents tense, anxious, irritable	14
Mother had a depressive illness; father schizoid, withdrawn, introverted	3
Mother obsessional, tense, anxious; father tense, anxious, irritable	3
Mother normal; father tense, anxious, irritable	3
Mother normal; father schizoid	3
Mother had a depressive illness; father tense, anxious, irritable	3
Mother detached, vague, schizoid; father tense, anxious, irritable	2
Mother tense, anxious, irritable; father schizoid, withdrawn, introverted	2
Mother tense, anxious, irritable; father normal	2
Mother had a depressive illness; father psychopathic	1
Mother hypomanic; father paranoid	1
Mother tense, anxious, irritable; father psychopathic	1
Both parents psychopathic	1
Mother over protective, withdrawn, vague; father normal	1
Mother had a depressive illness; father normal	1
Mother subnormal; father normal	1

In one case a maternal grandmother had a depressive illness but both parents were normal; in one case the mother was obsessional, tense and anxious while a paternal uncle had had a leucotomy; however, the nature of the illness was not known.

It will be seen in our series that the heredity in the case of psychotic children is heavily weighted. This is opposed to the views of Creak and Ini (1960) who did not think the attitudes or personality of the parents in their group very abnormal.

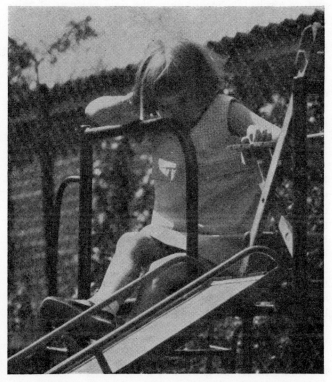

Figure 2. Typical withdrawn phase of the psychotic child.

On the other hand Goldfarb (1964) stresses the parental inadequacy as being of very great importance in the aetiology of the illness. He also stresses parental perplexity apparently concerning both their role in bringing up the children in general and also the methods of dealing with the deviant child. Again, Eisenberg and Kanner (1956) describe 'emotional frigidity' 'almost total absence of emotional warmth' in their series of parents. They also state that they attended to the physical needs of their children 'mechanically and on a schedule according to the rigid precepts of naive behaviourism applied with a vengeance'.

In twenty cases the children came from a very disturbed background. Commonly the child was rejected by the parents long before it became a disruptive influence in the household while overcrowding, quarrelling and tensions in the home occurred. In six cases the mother worked in a full-time job and the child was left in a nursery or in the care of neighbours.

ONSET AND AETIOLOGY

In our view there are two types of psychosis in childhood. One is reactive to extreme deprivation and emotional difficulties—the other type is present from birth. We prefer to call the type of psychosis which is present from birth as being *primary* (this being the syndrome originally described by Kanner) and the type which may show its onset from about the age of two as being *reactive*. In the primary type the intelligent mother will state that while feeding the baby at the breast when a few months old the child appeared to be looking beyond her and made no attempt to focus on the mother. At this early age she felt she was making no contact with the child.

Again, we are familiar with the mother's description of the child who is 'too good' and takes no notice of auditory or visual stimuli, will not turn its head when a sudden noise occurs or will not look at an object when brought near its cot or pram. Because of this the child is often thought to be deaf or blind while in many cases, far from being too good, the child is continually grizzly. Again, some mothers show their lack of warmth by stating that they never babbled to the child when feeding it as they felt this was a waste of time. These mothers would seem to exemplify Goldfarb's remarks that they attend to the children's physical needs in a mechanical way.

The relationship of mother and child may be compared to that of an actor and his audience—a positive, warm performance from the actor may get a response from even the coldest audience, whereas an unresponsive audience may freeze up all but the most brilliant actors. In this way a mother who would be adequate with a normal baby may be so discouraged by lack of response from a psychotic child that she gives up and withdraws. Consequently, a baby who might respond to a warm and positive mother, although it is already handicapped, fails to be roused.

The reactive type obviously comes on at a later age. Up to the age of onset the child is described as being normal if it has passed its milestones normally and, in some cases, may even have started to develop speech. The illness may be associated with extreme and severe deprivation. (This will be seen in the case of A.B. which is described later.) Alternatively, it may be associated with a severe trauma. Hospitalization of a child or of its mother for a prolonged period may produce a severe trauma. This is especially the case where the mother has been in hospital to have another baby; the new baby is then brought home for the first time. This happened with one of the children in our series who developed measles while the mother was in hospital. The child was sent away from home for some time while she was infectious and returned home after a prolonged period to find mother with a new baby and a rival.

Another child developed normally until about the age of

three when a large box of Guy Fawkes fireworks in the hall was inadvertently set alight and exploded. The child was petrified with fear, lost all its speech and showed the classical symptoms of psychosis. These children, who develop a reactive psychosis by withdrawing in this way, show the classical symptoms of the illness. These symptoms differ in no way from those occurring in a primary psychosis. Bowlby (1951) describes a patient who, when suddenly separated from its mother, becomes inert, listless and apathetic. Although these symptoms may be chiefly depressive in nature they show the child's reaction to a sudden and severe deprivation.

Obviously, all children do not react to deprivation or trauma in this way. It may well be that genetic factors play a part in that the premorbid personality of the child is such that it is extremely vulnerable to this type of trauma. At the moment no one can give an accurate aetiology of psychosis of childhood and biochemical, genetic, environmental and neurophysiological views have been propounded. In our opinion much more research is necessary into the aetiology of this illness. It would be of benefit and advantage to all those who are working with this problem to pool their ideas rather than to continue in watertight compartments as is happening at the present time.

In the uncomplicated psychotic group, physical aetiological factors were not as common as would be expected. During pregnancy there was a history of toxaemia in five cases, in one there was a history of severe influenza at the third month, while in one case there were rhesus factors present. Among the neonatal factors were three cases of prematurity, three of prolonged labour, three of anoxia, one of which was doubtful, and one case of jaundice. Again, there were few cases which gave a history of illness or physical trauma as aetiological factors. In one case there was a history of measles, one child fell down a flight of stairs but sustained no injury and one child was hit on the head with an iron bell; following this he was afraid of noise. In another child there was a dubious history of meningitis. Another child was immunized against whooping cough at nineteen months and suffered from severe anaphylactic shock.

Psychological traumata were not uncommon, as was seen in the child involved in the fireworks explosion, another who

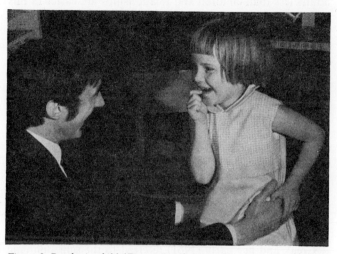

Figure 3. Psychotic child (Figure 2) relating with adult with whom she is familiar after being under treatment for some time.

fell into a reservoir and another who at eighteen months was on a railway platform when a train rushed through—the child became panic stricken. These are typical examples of the traumata found in these children. The different theories of causation are not necessarily contradictory. Like the old controversy between nature and nurture they may be supplementary to each other in that the end result is from an interaction between the two. Because of perceptual difficulties the child finds his or her environment very confusing and, as Goldfarb (1964) says, confused parents lead to a confused child. However, the child's behaviour may lead to the parents' confusion which in its turn makes the child worse and soon there is a vicious circle. The greater the innate handicap the more unpredictable the most normal environment becomes. Objects alter less than humans, and adults less than children and relationships are easier in this order. As the innate handicap becomes less, more abnormality in the environment is needed to produce symptoms. This could be a possible explanation of the better outlook for children with bad backgrounds and large emotional problems, as shown in this series.

DISCUSSION

In our series we have had two cases of juvenile schizophrenia in children aged ten who showed the classical symptoms of schizophrenia as seen in the adult. They exhibited auditory hallucinations, paranoid delusions, passivity feelings and thought disorder. This could in no way be confused with the illness which we are describing as psychosis in childhood.

Creak and her party (1961) referred to the schizophrenic syndrome of childhood and put forward their now well-known nine points as being diagnostic criteria.

In point (8) they talk of immobility as in katatonia and bizarre postures but these are rarely seen in psychoses of childhood. One does admittedly see mannerisms which are repeatedly carried out and withdrawal of a marked degree. In no way, however, do they resemble katatonia as seen in true schizophrenic states. In point (9) they give a background of serious retardation as one of their criteria and in our series we did not find severe subnormality as a common symptom.

PSYCHOLOGICAL TESTING

Twenty-one of the 66 cases were able to be tested formally and the results were as follows.

I.Q.	
I.Q. 120	1
I.Q. 115	1
I.Q. 110	4
I.Q. 100	2
I.Q. 95	1
I.Q. 90	5
I.Q. 85	3
I.Q. 75	1
I.Q. 70	1
I.Q. 60	2

In many children, however, it was felt that the I.Q. was not a true measure of their intelligence and that the result was an underestimation. Even among the untestable children it was apparent from their social behaviour and responses in the classroom that they were not functioning at a seriously retarded level. Wing (1966) states that the intelligence of the psychotic children varied from severely subnormal to above average but most showed at least some mental retardation and often it was severe. In our series the majority certainly did not show severe mental retardation although many of them, especially in the early stages of their stay, appeared to be functioning at a very low level due to the severely disturbed behaviour.

SYMPTOMATOLOGY IN THIS SERIES

In our series the following symptoms were found.

(1) *Withdrawal*—Withdrawal with consequent inability to make emotional relationships with other people, although their degree of this fluctuated and was not by any means constant. Again, in very withdrawn children separation from the parents often produced a further degree of disturbance. This can be shown by actual tears and distress,

loss of appetite and increased sleep disturbance. It is often impossible to make any rapport with these children in the early stages and their contact with reality is extremely tenuous. Some children are so withdrawn that they merge into the background and one is not conscious of their presence.

(2) *Visual and auditory avoidance*—These symptoms are, of course, extremely common and quite a number were referred because it was thought that they were deaf or blind. Many psychotic children either 'look through' the person, look beyond him or look at the ground. Many children with auditory avoidance are thought to be deaf and in our experience it may take weeks or even months of observation of these children before deafness can be excluded. Some of these children not only show no response to exceedingly loud auditory stimuli but even show no flicker of the eyelids when the stimulus occurs behind the head. In addition, these children are often seen sitting or walking with their hands tightly clasped over their ears as if they wished to exclude auditory contact with the outside world. Many children peer closely at objects and sniff them and lick them, while some children like feeling things with their fingers like a blind child.

(3) *Resistance to change*—This occurs from an early age. It may be partly due to this that the child becomes withdrawn and also shows marked anxiety when any change does occur in the environment. This resistance to change may be partly responsible for the food fads so commonly seen when the child is taken off the bottle or the breast and given a more solid diet.

Again, visual and auditory avoidance may also be the result of this resistance as the child does not wish to see or hear any change in the environment. This resistance may continue for a considerable time and only seem to diminish when the child becomes less withdrawn and begins to make better relationships with those in its environment. One child, when taken for a walk, became extremely anxious and disturbed when leaving the house but the increased anxiety did not occur on every occasion. Eventually, it was discovered that the boy was terrified of cars and it was only when he saw a car on leaving that he became so anxious. It was thought at first that this was due to change but obviously it was not. It may well be where a child is thought to be disturbed because of change that he is, in fact, disturbed by some object, the nature of which we are not aware.

We have observed that when some children are becoming less withdrawn and making more contact with their environment they become increasingly anxious and disturbed for some time. They also suffer from what would be described in adults as panic attacks.

(4) *Lack of response to other stimuli*—In addition to avoidance of visual and auditory stimuli, many of these children do not respond to tactile or painful stimuli. Although they do not respond to ordinary touching and, in many cases, dislike cuddling or physical contact with another being, it has been observed that tickling produces a response. Their reaction to this is one of delight and appropriate emotional responses occur in the form of giggling or even loud laughter. Some children when held upside down appear to react more normally both emotionally and in their relationships with other people. This also occurs in baths and paddling pools.

Many of these children lick themselves and it would appear that they are substituting primitive gustatory sensations for tactile ones. In addition, they often ignore painful stimuli and may burn themselves without any emotional response while they also tend to mutilate themselves by pinching, biting, and so on, without any apparent pain. One child under our care pulled off his toe nails and lined them up neatly under his bed apparently without suffering any pain. Another child clawed herself repeatedly until she produced a large open wound on her shoulder.

It may well be that these children have perceptual difficulties because of their abnormal reactions to almost any form of sensory stimulus. It may be that they are seeing objects in some distorted way. Sounds may be distorted in a like manner and in order to escape from these unpleasant stimuli they show avoidance and withdrawal. At the present time the nature of any such perceptual difficulties is not known and obviously such a theory must be purely speculative.

(5) *Speech difficulties*—In our series 48 children had no speech. In some cases speech had developed normally; then, following a trauma such as hospitalization, speech disappeared completely and often some years afterwards had not again developed. In other cases children showed echolalia and in the 18 children in our series who had some speech this was echolalic and meaningless.

Again, these children would use the third person when referring to themselves or would refer to themselves as 'you'. We have also seen children who refer to themselves by their christian names and then call the person talking to them by the same name. Some children have been observed to attempt to talk to their reflection in mirrors but will make no attempt to talk at other times. Obviously, failure to communicate is part of the child's withdrawal. However, it is difficult to understand why in some cases the child has no speech at all and in other cases only that of an echolalic type. Most of these children respond to rhythm and quite a high proportion are able to sing quite well and in tune. Williams (1968) states that speech development depends on various factors, three of which seem to be generally recognized. These are stimulation, frequency and the development of concepts.

Where children suffer from insufficient stimulation and are brought up in a culturally deprived background they tend to use language in a very restricted way. Not only are they lacking verbal stimulation but, in addition, stimulation by different types of games and play material, which seems to encourage various types of language, is also lacking. This may be due not only to a culturally deprived background but also to one or both parents being withdrawn and showing lack of warmth to, and interest in, the child. Williams states that a possible mechanism underlying the connections between language and other forms of behaviour is the formation of cross modal associations. Bartlett (1932) showed that we store and recall visual impressions largely according to the names we give them when first seeing them. More recent work has shown that even conditional responses are influenced by verbal associations. Thus, if a reflex has been established to the sound of a bell, it can be evoked by the word 'bell' and by a number of other words associated with it—Luria and Vinogradova (1959). Williams states that only in cases of organic cerebral dysfunction does the generalization of cross modal associations appear to be absent. It would, however, appear that in psychotic children a similar state of affairs occurs where there is no obvious organic brain damage.

The effects of frequency are obvious but the development of concept formation is more difficult and complicated. In order to apply the word 'table' to its appropriate object the child has to learn the exact features which make up a table. The word to begin with may be applied to many objects and it is only when he can distinguish the essential features of a table that he can use the word appropriately. He then finds the word 'table' can be used in an abstract sense—a table of figures, for instance. Apart from the fact that the psychotic child in many cases is deprived of learning speech because of lack of stimulation and frequency, there would appear to be difficulty in concept formation and absence of cross modal associations.

(6) *Mannerisms*—These children show many mannerisms. Spinning, rocking, and head rolling are commonly seen, while obsessional preoccupations with taps, arranging toys

and bricks in rows and various forms are also found. One child tore pieces of paper skilfully and quickly in an elaborate pattern which he repeated over and over. The pattern was mathematically exact on each occasion.

(7) *Obsessional preoccupations*—Several children had preoccupations with cleanliness and were very disturbed when any dirt was found on their clothing. Again, if another child upset the line of their bricks the child developed tantrums and became exceedingly anxious. Some children show this preoccupation with their own body, licking themselves, peering at their limbs as if they were not cognizant with their own body image. Some children would sit on the swing in the garden for hours swaying gently backwards and forwards. Again, it was not clear whether this was done for soporific or relaxing effect or was a stereotype.

(8) *Food fads*—Most of the children on admission showed marked food fads according to the parents—some of two or three years of age were still on the bottle. It was surprising, however, how quickly all these children, after being resident for a short time, overcame these fads and were on a normal diet.

(9) *Sleep disturbance*—These are common. The disturbances vary from difficulty in getting off to sleep to waking in the early hours and not going to sleep again. Waking in the night with what appeared to be night terrors in which they screamed and seemed to be terrified was also common. Some children who slept in dormitories tried to get into other children's beds. Whether this was done because they felt insecure and wanted human contact or whether they were doing this for some sexual reason was not clear. In some cases they attempted to get into the beds of children of the same sex, in others of the opposite sex.

(10) *Enuresis*—Enuresis was common among the children but after admission this cleared up fairly rapidly and recurred usually only when there was some emotional upset. Encopresis was not so common but did continue in some

70

cases and was accompanied by smearing faeces on themselves, other children and their toys.

(11) *Aggression and destructiveness*—Most psychotic children have no knowledge of real danger and will climb out of windows, literally play with fire and run into the road in front of traffic if allowed to do so. Many of these children show marked panic without any apparent external cause. Masturbation is not uncommon and is usually a sign of anxiety.

(12) *Kinaesthetic sense*—It has been observed that many of these children appear to have a well developed kinaes-thetic sense among the uncomplicated psychotic cases. These children often walk on their toes in a dainty manner, often reminiscent of ballet dancers. One child who previously would not ride his bicycle impetuously got on to it one day and rode it at speed through a gap with only a few inches to spare between a wall and his father's car. The father then reduced the gap and the child again rode the bicycle through it without mishap. This child was the child who tore the paper up so skilfully in an obsessional manner.

(13) *Physical appearance*—A point which we feel should be emphasized is that as a group psychotic children appear to be particularly attractive in looks. This, in view of the poor prognosis at the present time, makes the position so much sadder for their parents.

(1) CASE HISTORY—(X.Y.) PRIMARY TYPE

X.Y. is an example of primary psychosis of childhood. She was admitted in July, 1962 for investigation of her communication difficulties; she had been born in May, 1956.

The child had not babbled and at the age of three had a few words—'mum', 'look', and so on. Advice was sought at this time. The family history was negative apart from the fact that the mother was not very bright and a paternal uncle was deaf and dumb. The patient was the fifth child in a family of seven children—two boys and two girls were older than the patient, one boy and one girl younger. The remaining children were friendly, normal children and the home background was a happy one.

The pregnancy and confinement were normal, she passed her milestones a little early and was toilet trained from an early age. She was, however, fascinated by the lavatory chain and would spend long periods repeatedly pulling the the chain. From the age of two years she went around banging her head on doors and would rock herself in the cot until she moved it across the room. At times she showed tantrums, screamed and threw chairs about and also broke ornaments. At other times she played with the fire and threw clothing on it while she was preoccupied with milk or hot water bottles. She liked playing on swings and dressing up but became disinterested when given dolls. She was neat in the home and went around tidying things and became upset if she was thwarted. She had no idea of danger and, like so many psychotic children, she played with fire and would climb out of windows if allowed. She also carried around a cup and would take it to bed with her.

On admission she had no speech, was withdrawn, and showed visual and auditory avoidance. At times she was over active and destructive if frustrated. She was unco-operative, wandering around putting chairs in certain positions and showing aimless obsessional preoccupation.

Chromatography and EEG examination were normal but the child was myopic. She peered at objects closely, licked her clothes and was difficult over her diet. She was seen by our ophthalmologist, given glasses and appeared to hold her head up more readily. She did not show so much visual avoidance. Psychological testing (performance) showed her to have an I.Q. around 75 but this was probably an under-estimation. This child improved slowly and developed a certain amount of spontaneous speech. She showed more confidence especially after using her glasses. She recognized the names of other children, matched words and figures and copied simple shapes, pictures and letters. She also enjoyed all physical activities and made better relationships with the other children. She was transferred to Edith Edwards House School in July, 1963.

In May, 1968 she was reported as still being withdrawn and obsessional but fairly co-operative and joining in group activities. She responded well to music and was more interested in her surroundings. She also enjoyed physical training. This child is now aged 12 and the likelihood of her going into an ordinary educational establishment appears to be remote.

(2) CASE HISTORY—(A.B.) REACTIVE TYPE

A.B. was referred to our units in 1955, as she was thought to be deaf and subnormal. She was born in November, 1950 and came from a disturbed home background—the mother was rather cold emotionally, had difficulty in mixing and was immature. The father was also immature and at the time of the patient's admission there was a boy of 13 months who was quite normal.

During the pregnancy the mother had had no specific illness but suffered from malaise. Prior to this pregnancy she had had several miscarriages. The baby had been born in hospital, and the mother complained that she was sent home ill and was ill at home with septicaemia because 'they left the afterbirth in'. Since A.B.'s birth there had been trouble with her feeding, she was sick every day and the mother undertook long journeys to a welfare clinic which upset her.

The child's health improved but the sickness then recurred and the parents thought the child deliberately brought on the vomiting to make things awkward for them. She then went to a local day nursery but the mother felt they did not understand the child. At this time the child developed odd postures and would remain in these positions, head thrown back, eyes half shut, arms akimbo, for two to three hours. The child was wet and dirty and smeared faeces on the stairs. She had no speech at all. The maternal grandmother talked to the child 'as if she were a cat' and she was not allowed to play with the younger child. The parents said they had lost all their friends as a result of having an abnormal child.

On admission she showed no hearing loss, and EEG examination was normal. She was, however, extremely destructive, tearing up her clothing, was wet and dirty and at times stood for long periods completely withdrawn. She was unable to dress herself and any break in routine made her more difficult and negativistic. At times she had screaming attacks or played with her fingers, while at other times she was tearful. She had some comprehension of speech on admission. Her verbal I.Q. was 71 and performance I.Q. 106.

This child remained in our units for nearly four years as it was impossible to place her in either a suitable hospital or school. She gradually settled down, made social progress and was sent to a nursery school in Sutton for half a day daily where she made rapid strides. Her speech improved rapidly but she remained rather peevish and attention seeking. Her mood improved, she became a happy, helpful child and in 1959 she went to a residential special school for maladjusted children. She again improved scholastically but was still rejected by her parents and the headmistress of the school suggested a social worker might visit her home. This was arranged but the social worker was also rejected by the parents. She then went to a secondary modern school and did quite well.

In a recent communication from her mother (May, 1968) the mother stated that the girl, nearly 18 years of age, was training to be a punch card operator and earning over £10 per week. She was fitting well into the family, read science fiction and thrillers and wrote simple letters. She has difficulty in pronouncing and remembering long words, but did take a great interest in her appearance. In a photograph enclosed by her mother she looked an attractive young girl. Her mother stated that from 14 to 15 the patient seemed to live in a dream world and was unable to tell the truth; this coincided with the onset of menstruation. It would appear from the mother's description that A.B. is now a reasonably normal girl who is accepted by the family.

PSYCHOTIC AND BRAIN DAMAGED

In the psychotic and brain damaged group there were thirteen patients of whom ten were male and three were female.

AGE OF PARENTS

There was nothing significant in the ages of the parents apart from the fact that the father in one case was 46 and two mothers were aged 36 and 35 respectively.

HEREDITY

The family history was, however, significant in that in four cases both parents showed psychiatric symptoms and in four other cases one parent (the father) was abnormal. Where both parents showed abnormalities these were as follows.

(1) Father and mother tense and irritable.
(2) Mother tense and paranoid; father immature and depressed.
(3) Father highly strung, irritable and impatient; mother chronic neurotic.
(4) Mother highly strung and irritable; father schizoid, withdrawn and cold.

75

In the remaining four cases the fathers' symptoms were respectively as follows.

(1) Tense, anxious and schizoid.
(2) Authoritarian, alcoholic, unstable and rejected child.
(3) Schizophrenia while pgm was eccentric and pgf was a pyknic, moody person.
(4) Withdrawn and schizoid.

ENVIRONMENTAL FACTORS

In three cases there were tension and quarrelling in the home; in one case in addition the family lived in a caravan, moved about and there was no security, in a third case the child was illegitimate. As in the uncomplicated group of psychotic children, there was no significance in the position in the family of the disturbed child.

AETIOLOGICAL FACTORS

In two cases there was a history of toxaemia of pregnancy, one child was ten weeks premature and in one case there was a prolonged and difficult labour. Three patients suffered from neonatal jaundice and one from cyanosis. Three gave a history of measles and three of gastro-enteritis. One child at the age of thirteen months pulled a hall stand on to himself and suffered a fractured nose and cuts over the occipital and parietal areas. However, there was no evidence of a fractured skull.

PHYSICAL FINDINGS

Neurological signs were not common but ataxia hypotonia with high stepping gait, hyperactivity and spatial difficulties were found in six patients. Four gave a history of grand mal attacks and in ten of these patients the EEG's were abnormal. Fits did not occur in the uncomplicated psychotic children. Formal intelligence testing was only possible in five cases and these children had I.Q.s of 116, 100 (2), 77 and 60 respectively.

SYMPTOMATOLOGY

Five children had no speech at all. One had lost it at the age of two and a half years after being hospitalized while the other four had some indistinct words and also showed echolalia. In addition to the withdrawal and visual and auditory avoidance, these children were hyperkinetic to a marked degree and also had spatial difficulties.

CASE HISTORY—(D.E.) PSYCHOTIC WITH BRAIN DAMAGE

D.E. was a boy who was admitted to our units in August, 1963 because of behavioural problems and lack of communication. He was born in January, 1957 and his father was a highly strung, quick tempered Chinaman who frequently hit the children; the mother was a healthy woman who had become anxious over the child's condition. There was another boy of ten who was withdrawn, secretive and a poor mixer and a boy of eight who was mischievous and always in trouble. There were no prenatal or perinatal factors but he was jaundiced for two weeks after birth. His milestones were slightly delayed, he babbled and had a few simple words such as 'mum' and 'dad'. He was toilet trained from the age of four, was a poor eater but did feed himself. He had been investigated for deafness and this had been excluded. His previous medical history showed no significant illnesses.

The child looked an Oriental due to his Chinese ancestry. His head was flattened in the occipital region, he had a left internal strabismus and blue hands with spatulate, stubby fingers. This made fine movements difficult. He was withdrawn, did not relate with either children or adults, made sucking noises and took no notice of simple commands. Because of his fingers being fat and wrinkled and looking like a bunch of bananas he used his thumb and second fingers to manipulate things but his movements were clumsy. He slept badly, was restless at nights and got into other children's beds. He was a messy eater and became dirty in his habits, using the playroom floor for urinating and defaecating.

He still only had a few words, his comprehension was good but he had difficulty in writing and drawing because of his 'sausage like' fingers—as a result he became frustrated, screamed and was violent. He recognized pictures, numbers and matched objects well. His I.Q. was 118 and his EEG showed a definite left sided abnormality. At times his behaviour became so uncontrolled that it was necessary to give him largactil mg 75 *mane* and mg 50 *nocte* which was repeated if necessary. He settled down quite well and was transferred after three months to our house in Sutton. Eventually he was transferred to Edith Edward's House School in July, 1964. He showed no interest in other children but liked physical contact and on several occasions was found asleep in other children's beds. He was hyperactive, turning somersaults and doing other acrobatic tricks. He showed many obsessional traits, such as being afraid of anything generating heat. His bathwater had to be lukewarm and he would not venture near a radiator until someone had tested the warmth. He began to smell objects which he did not recognize as a means of finding out what they were. He enjoyed doing puzzles and using constructional play material.

By 1965 he had begun to read but still had little spontaneous speech. His memory was extremely good and he recognized numbers up to 100. However, he still made little contact with other children but his relationship with adults was fairly good. During this time he was also receiving speech therapy and showed marked interest in imitating speech sounds and, later, words. He resented change and still became frustrated by his poor writing skill. However, by June, 1966 he was more integrated in the group and less withdrawn. He eventually was sent to a Rudolf Steiner School where he is making slow progress.

PSYCHOTIC AND DEAF

In the psychotic and deaf group there were ten patients of whom six were male and four were female.

PARENTAL AGE

Parental age was only significant in three children. One child had a father of 41, and the mother was 38. In another patient the mother's age was 43 and the father's 42. In one other case the father's age was 38. Again, there was nothing significant about the child's position in the family.

HEREDITY

In the group of psychotic and brain damaged children it is noteworthy that more *fathers* showed neurotic symptoms; in this group the preponderance was among the *mothers*. In five cases the patients' mother showed psychiatric symptoms. These were subnormality, subnormality with neuroticism, depressive illness, neurosis and stammering in the mother and maternal grandmother.

ENVIRONMENTAL FACTORS

Two children were illegitimate and one was completely rejected by the parents.

AETIOLOGICAL FACTORS

In one case there was a history of toxaemia and, in another, rubella in pregnancy and one gave a history of a long and difficult labour. In one patient there was a history of postnatal cyanosis and in a fifth patient there was a history of jaundice.

SPEECH AND PSYCHOLOGICAL TESTING

As would be expected with children with the dual handicap of psychosis and deafness, none of these children had any speech at all and all were untestable to formal psychological testing. It was, however, only after long periods of observation that a decision could be made that these children were at least of average intelligence and were deaf.

SYMPTOMATOLOGY

Obviously, these children were extremely withdrawn and again showed many of the symptoms of uncomplicated psychosis. They resented change, showed obsessional traits, could not make relationships and showed bizarre mannerisms. These included flicking things, licking objects and in some cases a tendency to self-mutilation. In none of these children was there a history of fits.

CAUSES OF DEAFNESS

The cause of the deafness was not clear in some of the patients but the following were found as causal factors.

Toxaemia of pregnancy	1
Rubella in pregnancy	1
Neonatal jaundice	1
Neonatal cyanosis	1
Meningitis	1
Measles	1

CASE HISTORIES—(F.G. AND H.J.) PSYCHOTIC WITH DEAFNESS

F.G.—Deaf psychotic

This child was born in May, 1949 and admitted in February, 1957 having been referred from the Maudsley Hospital. The reason for his referral was the fact that he had been excluded from a school for the deaf because of his disruptive behaviour. There was only one significant point in the family history. In taking a history from the mother who was aged 35 at the time of F.G.'s birth, she was found to have been reserved in manner and had a wariness which made conversation difficult. She was also tense and anxious.

An independent witness, however, stated that the mother was always devoted to the patient and took a great interest in him. At the time that F.G.'s behavioural difficulties started she was to have another child who is a boy now aged three. There were no prenatal, perinatal, or postnatal factors but at the age of one year he began to have screaming fits at night which later changed into outbursts of wild laughter. He was always a noisy restless child who seemed to require less sleep than most children. At fourteen months he underwent an operation for intussusception but this did not appear to have affected him adversely. At eighteen months deafness was diagnosed and the mother attempted to teach the child with the aid of a correspondence course. According to her the immediate response was gratifying and he learned to identify objects, to write simple letters and to lip read simple directions. The mother thinks she may have attempted to push him too hard but there was a close relationship between them apart from meal times. There were frequent scenes, then he would go for days without food and the process of making him eat became a wearisome battle. His mother would forcibly hold the boy down while she pushed spoonfuls of mashed food into his resisting mouth. It seemed that the feeding difficulties assumed unreasonable proportions in the mother's mind.

Early in his fourth year he showed a marked and sudden change in his behaviour. He lost all desire to learn, he became solitary, self-absorbed and developed the habits of head rocking and masturbation. The mother sensed a barrier between the child and herself which she could not overcome. Shortly afterwards, the child was admitted to a residential school for the deaf where he remained for three years. He was then described as living in a world of his own, refusing to mix with his group, playing games on his own and showing extreme restlessness. He had attacks of head rolling, laughed and smiled to himself and at times had outbursts of wild laughter. He was tidy, able to dress himself and was toilet trained. He obeyed instructions, was never destructive but slept badly at night.

He occupied himself with jig-saws and mechanical puzzles and was able to add numbers up to 14. He also wrote clearly but was only able to copy in drawing. Recently he developed preoccupations with walls, running to them, pointing at them and being destructive with them. He showed other obsessional preoccupations in that he covered the heads of screws attached to taps with paper and played with the electric lights. When he was frustrated he developed temper tantrums lasting up to three quarters of an hour. He was right handed, prone to spells of overactivity and was restless before going to sleep and during sleep. He ate well now, had no speech but a high pitched whine most of the time. He was easily frustrated, made no relationships with other children and indulged in frequent masturbation. He enjoyed physical contact while his I.Q. was in the region of 118.

While an inpatient in our units his behaviour remained much the same but communication was established with him by means of reading and written commands. However, he did not communicate at all except by an occasional questioning look or leading someone by the hand. He showed elaborate twiddling movements of the fingers and a rather Peter Pan like dance when approaching anything which interested him.

EEG examination was within normal limits, his deafness was severe although an audiogram could not be obtained. In view of his I.Q. of 118, it was felt he should go to a Rudolf Steiner School and he did so in 1959. He attended a deaf class, made attempts to lip read, understood gestures and became more co-operative and helpful. He was still, however, withdrawn at times and would spend hours with jig-saw puzzles but his tantrums and screaming attacks were much less frequent. In May, 1968 he was in much the same state.

H.J.—Deaf psychotic

This child was born in May, 1957. He was admitted to our units in August, 1964 having been referred by a local authority because of behavioural problems and exclusion from school. He was the second of five children, three boys and two girls; the eldest child, a boy, was also deaf, as was the youngest, a girl. The oldest is in Exeter School for the Deaf and is doing quite well. He uses a hearing aid, has little speech as yet, and only a small amount of lip reading. The girl of fourteen months uses a hearing aid and is apparently quite normal. A paternal uncle had three children, two of whom are at residential deaf schools. One child is severely deaf and one child is partially deaf with a fair amount of speech. Both parents were hearing people and the father, who was aged 34, was a disturbed, suspicious man.

The pregnancy and confinement were normal but there was a possibility that the patient was cyanosed at birth. He was somewhat slow in passing his milestones, never babbled and was not clean until about the age of six.

On admission he showed visual avoidance, was withdrawn and made no relationships either with children or adults. He had no speech, made peculiar grunts indicative of pleasure and was quite skilful in doing jig-saw puzzles. He refused to use his hearing aid and at times was vicious and aggressive towards other children. He showed extensive pica from an early age and has been preoccupied with wheels from at least two and a half years. He also showed pre-occupation with putting together blocks and had short tantrums when frustrated in doing this. He appeared to be a compulsive masturbator, was destructive and showed mannerisms of his hands especially when excited. Chromatography and EEG examination were normal and he showed a performance test of 98. He remained in the unit until September, 1966 and during this time he showed considerable improvement. He became more disciplined but at times was very frustrated and cried with temper. He improved socially, was clean, fed himself and was much less withdrawn. He became skilful with constructional toys, painting and his imaginative play was quite good. He accepted routine quite well and discipline also.

The child remained with us for two years as it was felt he should be found a suitable school or hospital in view of his level of intelligence. Unfortunately, this was not possible and he has now been admitted to a subnormal institution.

This child showed two distinct but interacting causes for his inability to communicate—a profound genetic deafness and the psychotic syndrome of childhood. The psychotic syndrome of childhood was definitely remitting but his difficulty with symbols and visual avoidance made communication either by learning to read or to lip read virtually impossible. Communication with him was registered only if he gestured which he (as with psychotic children) rarely did.

This child is typical of many psychotic deaf children of average intelligence who require therapeutic education in a special unit, either school or hospital, of which there is none at the present time.

Placement

This type of child must of necessity at present be relegated to a training centre or institution for subnormals where obviously any possible chance of help is negligible. This is not because one decries such units but because a child of this type needs to be in a unit where the staff is specially trained in coping with both deaf and psychotic children as both handicaps are present. In addition to this, the ratio of staff to patients must be high.

CASE HISTORY—(L.M.) DEAF PSYCHOTIC AND BRAIN DAMAGE

This little girl, who was born in September, 1956, was admitted in January, 1965 and had been referred by a school medical officer. She was to be excluded from Margate School for the Deaf where she had been for two and a half years, mainly because of behavioural problems and the fact that she had made no social or educational progress.

The family history was negative, the patient was the third of four children; the other three were normal boys. A fifth baby died at six days, having been premature.

The confinement had been difficult. There had been a delay of twelve hours at the actual birth and cerebral anoxia was suspected. The child was born with a bruised forehead, and oedematous orbits. She had shown some delay in passing her milestones but apparently began to babble at ten months. She had bladder and bowel control at four and a half years and at two and a half years she was diagnosed as being severely deaf. From three to four years she received speech therapy twice a week until her admission to school.

On admission she showed periods of withdrawal, obsessional preoccupations with feeling clothes and hair and at times she gesticulated at imaginary audiences as if she were visually hallucinated. She smiled to herself, would stroke fluffy clothing for long periods, and at times she suffered from periodic outbursts of violence. At times her periods of withdrawal were similar to trance-like states but at times she was able to relate to other people fairly well. She attempted to communicate by primitive sign language. During her violent episodes, which were apparently unprovoked, she would bite, scratch or hit out at the nearest bystander. She had at first insisted on being dressed as a boy and on one occasion cut off her hair. Later she showed a more overt sexuality by attempting to get any observer to lie down and attempt to make them lie close to her.

Chromatography was negative while a number of EEG's were carried out under sedation. These showed evidence of right sided brain damage while she did not respond to very loud noises on the EEG. She showed areas of intelligence function well above her chronological age (nine) and on the W.I.S.C. grading she produced a response equivalent in mental age to a child aged eleven and a half years. She showed no neurological signs and was investigated at the National Hospital, Queen Square, London, W.C. X-ray of the skull and chest were normal, an air encephalogram was normal and all biochemical investigations were normal.

FOLLOW-UP

An attempt was made to follow up all the psychotic children by letter. Unfortunately, in many cases either no reply was received or the letters were returned and there was no other means of contacting the parents. Follow-up reports were received from 61 parents relating to 39 male and 22 female patients. Six patients (three female and three male) had improved considerably. In all these cases the conditions were reactive psychoses and in no case of primary psychosis had the child shown any marked improvement— in short, although the children or adolescents were by now less withdrawn, had developed a certain amount of speech and were more amenable generally, they were still unable to attend ordinary educational establishments or live in the community and undertake any form of work.

One girl aged thirteen and a half who attends a secondary modern school has fluent speech, is in the correct form for her age but in the lowest stream. A year ago she was second in her form but her work fluctuates considerably. She still has difficulty in mixing and is described by her parents as 'not wishing to grow up'. She frequently says things like 'everyday life is boring' and 'phantasy is much more interesting and exciting'. Another girl of fifteen is at an ordinary school and apparently doing quite well while the third girl whose case was described (*see* pp. 73–75) is learning to be a punch card operator. Two boys are still at school and doing quite well. Another boy is working as a market gardener and living in a hostel. These children appear to have made the best adjustments but, even so, they could not be described as being completely normal.

Of the children suffering from primary psychoses 23 had developed speech varying from six to 150 words, three had a few sentences. Thirteen were said to be less withdrawn although their ability to make relationships with other people was very limited.

PROGNOSTIC CRITERIA

In our view there are no clinical criteria on which an accurate prognosis can be based. For instance, the children who had a few words at an early age did no better than those who had no speech at all. Those children in the higher ranges of I.Q.s again did no better than those in the lower ranges.

Absence or presence of obsessional features, marked dislike of change, visual or auditory avoidance or the degree of withdrawal did not seem to affect the prognosis in any way.

LACK OF FACILITIES

Follow-up letters were received from 61 parents and of these six children (9·1 per cent) had made a reasonable adjustment. The remainder of the children who, because of their age, had to leave the special units where they were receiving treatment are now in subnormal or mental hospitals or training centres if they are unable to remain at home.

It is appalling at the present time that when these children become adolescents there are no special units to which they can go. At the moment, if institutional treatment is necessary, they have to go to subnormal or mental hospitals where they mix with the other patients. No special observation or training is given to them apart from that provided for the other patients. In our opinion it is essential that special hostels should be provided for these patients. This will ensure further research on them and will also provide the opportunity of training them for some sort of routine job in a sheltered environment.

At the moment the outlook for recovery for psychotic children is extremely gloomy. In most units where these children are given what we would like to call 'therapeutic education' in the early stages almost individual education would appear to be necessary. Eventually it is hoped that when the child learns to make relations with other children and adults they can then be taught in small groups. It must be emphasized that in our experience any semblance of a hospital environment is absolutely wrong in trying to treat these children. This is because we have found that when children have been transferred for some time to a hospital environment, they have regressed considerably even when they have had a considerable time in the new environment in which to settle down.

DISCUSSION

Again, opinion is divided as to whether these children should live in a completely permissive environment or in a strictly disciplinarian one. It is obvious in the early days of a child's stay in a unit that permissiveness should be allowed to a great degree and then tempered with discipline as the child settles down and learns to make relationships with other children and adults. Again, there is no unanimity among psychiatrists as to whether these children should be treated in residential or day units. Probably neither is right for all and the correct way varies as with normal children.

Obviously, residential treatment would be recommended of necessity where there is no day unit for such children within a reasonable distance of the home. Again, where the family background is extremely disturbed, residential care should be recommended. Where the family is at breaking point in trying to cope with a psychotic child or where normal children in the family are suffering, residential care must be recommended.

Even when removal from home is advised contact with the home must be maintained, especially where the child appears to be fretting for the parents. Visits should be encouraged unless the child is too disturbed after being visited. Occasional weekends, half-term holidays and school holidays should also be spent at home by the children. It is important that the parents must be encouraged to accept their share of the responsibility and also take part in the general welfare of the child. Some parents reject the child completely and are anxious to obtain residential care in order that they may lead an unhampered social life. Some parents with children in residential care show no interest whatever in them. In families such as these, child and parent are better apart where there seems no hope of improving the parent-child relationship. It is obvious that the child is better off in a residential unit in such a case but an important aspect in dealing with such parents is to see them frequently (either individually or in groups) so that their attitude to the child may be altered.

Dr. Minski is in charge of the Lindens Special School at Saint Ebba's Hospital, Epsom, run by the Surrey County Council for severely disturbed children by Mrs. Barbara Furneaux. Here the children can attend the school from 9 a.m. to 3 p.m. daily and transportation to and from home is provided by the local authority. All of the children live in the county. Therefore, the parents are accessible to the school and to the psychiatrist and, in fact, they are encouraged to attend daily at the school if they so wish. Where it is found that the home situation is impossible, there are a few residential places to which the child can be admitted. On the whole, however, an attempt is made to keep the child as a day boarder so that continuity with the parents and other members of the family is maintained.

In our opinion and experience there is a place for these children in both day and residential units. In fact, the same child may benefit by residential care at one period and by day care at another. With many children a temporary residence may be advisable for the following reasons.

(1) To give parents a rest from the child.

(2) To give the child a rest from the parents and give both a time of unemotional re-adjustment when they are not too involved with each other.

(3) To give opportunity for fuller assessment of child in a neutral environment.

(4) To provide time to help parents to understand the situation better and be given advice and practical demonstrations on handling.

We have found children who, on admission to our units, are more disturbed on leaving their parents and are obviously fretting while they are in our units. Again, we have seen in some cases that when the child goes home for the weekend and returns to the unit, it is fretful, sleeps badly and becomes quieter (obviously homesick and depressed). We have, however, only seen two children who have had to be returned home as they were obviously so upset that we felt they should.

O'Gorman (1967) states that it will often be advisable to remove the child from the incompatible family situation and place him in hospital. He does stress that this should be done gradually and that complete loss of contact between mother and child is nearly always undesirable. With some cases where parents are very good and the child is not too disruptive an element or where relationship between parents and the child is in a critical stage of development, it may be important that the child should live at home. Without doubt there seems to be a place for both types of treatment and, ideally, it should be possible to have access to short stay beds in times of emergency or for periods of rest in those children who remain at home.

OPERANT CONDITIONING

About three years ago at Belmont Hospital, Humphery was able to initiate operant conditioning on a research grant. This was continued also on a research basis by Evans under clinical supervision.

Operant conditioning is a form of behaviour therapy. The basis is that if behaviour is followed by something which the patient likes, such as attention, food or a smile, then the behaviour will tend to be repeated. Therefore, behaviour which is rewarded will tend to increase whereas behaviour which is punished will tend to be eliminated. For instance, at meal times a child is given its food only if it uses a knife and fork, or a sweet only if it washes its hands and face before the meal. A child may only be given a sweet if it says 'please' or 'thank you'. Verbal behaviour is bound to increase as it is positively reinforced. Help, of course, must be given to the child and encouragement is an important aspect.

Normal behaviour other than verbal can also be established by the proper use of positive reinforcement. A child can be taught with pieces of chocolate and much encouragement to do up his buttons or dress himself. The child must, however, be given the opportunity to perform the appropriate behaviour before it can be established through positive reinforcement. This demands much patience on the part of the staff. The child can be taught through positive reinforcement to set the table, bathe himself, play with others, and, in fact, indulge in any normal behaviour. The reinforcement must be used quickly and consistently upon the performance of normal behaviour. An attempt to eliminate abnormal behaviour can be made by negative reinforcement, that is, by punishment. This does not mean slapping the child or using an electric shock. It may mean simply not giving the child what he wants if he is mute or ignoring temper tantrums or crying fits. It may mean isolating the child if he is aggressive and hits another child. Again, these negative reinforcements must be used consistently and immediately following abnormal behaviour.

One does not, however, want the child to feel he is rejected and disliked. Every time a negative reinforcement is given the opportunity of using a positive reinforcement should be taken. Thus, when he stops crying he should be cuddled or given the object which he wants. This switching from negative reinforcement for abnormal behaviour to positive reinforcement for normal behaviour is like a see-saw. With this combination of rewards and punishment the child may develop a good relationship with members of the staff.

Operant conditioning is only a more systematic form of the methods used by anyone who is 'good at bringing up children'. Consistency is more important for these children than normal children so that 'they know where they are'.

8—General Observations

An analysis of 474 children with verbal communication difficulties shows that these may be due to the following.

(1) Subnormality.
(2) Deafness.
(3) Emotional disturbance.
(4) Aphasia.
(5) Brain damage.
(6) Psychosis.

CAUSES OF NON-COMMUNICATION

It has been seen that in quite a number of children the difficulties are due to a multiplicity of causes. This is particularly true in cases of subnormality with emotional difficulties, subnormality and deafness, aphasia and deafness, psychosis with deafness and/or brain damage.

Subnormality may be due to a variety of causes ranging from illness or toxic factors in pregnancy to illness in the early years of life. Obviously, in a number of cases genetic factors are of the utmost importance. We would, however, like to stress the giving of drugs to pregnant mothers as in many cases these are exhibited too lightly or carelessly. Thus, antidepressant drugs are given freely by some psychiatrists and the toxic effects of these drugs on the foetus are not really understood. Again, pregnant mothers who are epileptic continue to take a wide variety of anticonvulsant drugs during the pregnancy and often in quite large doses. Here again, the effects of the drugs on the foetus have not been determined.

Mauser and colleagues (1968) treated twelve pregnant women with 30–120 mg phenobarbitone for two weeks or longer prior to delivery. Subsequently, concentrations of serum-bilirubin in their offspring and in sixteen control babies were compared during the first four days of life. Serum-bilirubin levels were significantly lower in babies of treated mothers and the data suggests that phenobarbitone received during pregnancy decreased the concentration of neonatal serum-bilirubin. This suggests that phenobarbitone administered in the last two weeks of pregnancy may reduce the risk of neonatal jaundice but the effects of other anticonvulsant drugs on the foetus are not really known.

The effects of antibiotics are also not fully understood and the number of drugs given freely to pregnant mothers in our opinion should be controlled. Macaulay and Watson (1967) refer to hypernatraemia as a cause of brain damage in infants.

One-hundred-and-twenty-two children out of 695 were hypernatraemic and of these 47 were suffering from diarrhoeal diseases, 13 had pneumonia, and 27 had more than one disorder. In 35 the diagnoses ranged from meningitis to appendix abscess.

The age range varied from one day to two years three months and the minimal interval of follow-up from the date of admission was eighteen months. The longest was eight years. Reliable information was available about the fate of 114 of the 122 children. In 33 of the 114 brain damage was demonstrated at necropsy or inferred from clinical evidence.

Undoubted association between hypernatraemia and brain damage may indicate either a liability to cerebral damage from the electrolyte disturbance or the possibility of hypernatraemia being of neurogenic origin. This is the opinion of the authors. The authors also stress the fact that prevention presents better hope of reducing its incidence than treatment of established hypernatraemia. It is hoped that further research will be undertaken on these lines.

It would appear at the present time that too little money is available for research into the causes of subnormality. If sufficient funds were available something might be done in preventing many cases of subnormality which should not be allowed to occur. There are not enough facilities in the form of clinics where the parents of subnormal children can receive support and guidance in coping with these handi-capped children and more money should be spent on these facilities. Emotional difficulties are more common among deaf children in the higher levels of intelligence. This is perhaps to be expected as they have more insight into their inability to communicate and in this way they become more frustrated and disturbed.

There is one point we would like to emphasize. Where a deaf child of average intelligence cannot learn by lip reading, the child is, in our experience, incapable of learning in this way due to a specific language difficulty as a result of brain damage. In order to help the frustrations of these children the only method of communication is by means of 'signing' and these children should be taught accordingly. In a recent report from the Department of Education and Science they agree implicitly that signing and finger spelling should be used as an aid to communication. Surely communication by some means is better than no means of communication at all. Where a child is definitely shown to be deaf at an early age it should be fitted with a hearing aid at once, if its hearing is likely to benefit from the use of one. Rejection of the aid is less likely to occur and the child is more likely to become adapted to sound at an early age than when this is left until later in life. Apart from rejection of an aid because of physical discomfort (due to a badly fitting mould) rejection may occur as a result of too much amplification. This can also produce mental discomfort. It is in problems arising in this way that a stay at a hostel (for example, the hostel at Ealing) would benefit mothers. Here they can be reassured about the use of a hearing aid and the difficulties arising therefrom. Apart from this the parents of any handicapped family require support and advice in coping with such a child and more clinics should be available for this purpose.

We would like to stress that many deaf children show emotional difficulties which are undiagnosed. Obviously, the child who is disturbed in a positive way will be readily diagnosed—the passive and withdrawn child who sits in a classroom without causing any disturbance may well pass unnoticed. For this reason all audiology units should have a child psychiatrist attached to them. In fact, the services of a team consisting of psychiatrist, psychologist, social worker, pediatrician and E.N.T. specialist are really essential.

In assessing all children where the nature of the handicap is not obvious, continual observation over a prolonged period in a residential unit is essential. The true condition often only unfolds itself after such a period of observation. This period of observation may make all the difference in that a child may often be regarded as educable instead of being regarded as ineducable. For instance, it was only the result of such observation that the child whose case was illustrated on pp. 46–47, who had aphasia, deafness and emotional difficulties was able to be correctly diagnosed. It took almost eighteen months to make the diagnosis but the child is now doing well in a small class in a partially hearing school. In our view this would not have been possible if a hurried diagnosis on an outpatient basis had been attempted.

At the present time, however, there are too few units for assessment purposes as well as places for the children who need therapeutic education. There is also an urgent need for more beds for disturbed children and more units for psychotic children. Although we have presented a gloomy picture regarding the prognosis for psychotic children, we do not wish it to be inferred that work both from the research and therapeutic aspects should be abandoned. We hope that the people working in these units for psychotic children will pool their ideas and results and not work in watertight compartments. In this way it is hoped that workers in this field will develop a unified approach to this most difficult problem.

The placement of children in special units or schools is, unfortunately, extremely difficult. For instance, an aphasic child who is emotionally disturbed is very often rejected by the schools because of the emotional disturbance. If one then attempts to obtain the child's admission to a school for maladjusted children, the child is again rejected because of lack of speech. Again such a child may have multiple handicaps including defective vision, deafness, aphasia and emotional difficulties. This is particularly true with rubella children. It is almost impossible to place such a child for educational and treatment purposes. Schools for the educationally subnormal child will not accept children who have speech disorders—schools dealing with speech disorders will not accept educationally subnormal children because they are regarded as being too low in the intellectual scale. These are practical difficulties which have repeatedly occurred with us in trying to place children who have passed through our units.

In our opinion it would be much more practical to have units or small classes which accept children with multiple handicaps as, at the present time, there is too much specialization in these schools. Many children at present fall between 'two schools'. It is regrettable that education authorities are not more far seeing and do not set up multipurpose schools for the handicapped child.

In treating psychotic children it has been our practice to avoid the use of drugs as much as possible. In a number of cases, however, it has been necessary to use drugs to contain the children for a time and also to tide them over some sudden crisis. These have consisted mainly of chlorpromazine stelazine, fentazin and haliperidol with in some cases Syr.tricloryl at night. These children appear to have an abnormal tolerance to drugs. When they are exhibited to these children in adult doses the effects on the children are minimal and very transient.

One child who went home for some days was taking Syr. tricloryl 12 ml *nocte* and his parents were given a 120 ml bottle to take with them. They were given a warning not to allow the child to have access to the bottle which they unfortunately did and he swallowed the contents at one session. His parents telephoned the unit in great distress and they were told to take the child to the casualty department of a nearby hospital. The child showed no ill effects from the large dose of Syr.tricloryl and, in fact, was hardly drowsy. This is an extreme example of the resistance which psychotic children show towards drugs.

We would like to emphasize again the urgent need for more classes for aphasic children and also the need for more small classes for brain damaged children of average or above average intelligence. At the present time, these are sadly lacking. In some areas there is a most acute shortage of speech therapists and speech therapy available to children. We would again like to stress the overcrowding and understaffing in many of the subnormal hospitals. Many children, if facilities in hostels were available, would be able to live outside of hospitals. To a degree this would ease the overcrowding.

Even so, the ratio of patients to staff would still be excessive. In our view most of the children in subnormal hospitals do not require nursing but affection and security. We see no reason to have nurses in uniforms. Kindly girls and women who dress like the children's mothers at home, possibly with a nylon overall or apron acting as mother substitutes, would be more to the point. There is no real necessity for doctors to walk around their wards in white coats which are often terrifying to the children. In our view, in dealing with all groups of disturbed children, the hospital atmosphere should be removed as far as possible and the children should be treated in a more 'homelike' atmosphere.

We dislike the name 'child guidance clinic' and would prefer the name 'child health clinic'. In any case, the name is a misnomer. Some parents object to taking their children to such a clinic, especially where they feel guilty and blame themselves for the child's emotional difficulties. We would like to see these clinics more closely linked with general and paediatric hospitals. In addition, day units should be provided so that mother and child can attend two or three times weekly. At the present time they are often only able to attend about once a month which is obviously most unsatisfactory in attempting to solve the problem. We have also mentioned the importance of clinics at which the parents of any handicapped child can receive support and guidance. At the present time, these exist only in a very few areas and more could be set up without any great financial expense.

We would also like to see antenatal clinics offering help in the psychological and emotional field to expectant mothers. The attitude of the mother to the child could in this way be helped considerably. For instance, over protection and unconscious rejection could be avoided. The mother who shows little warmth to her child because of its make-up might be helped; she could also be instructed about babbling and talking to the child when feeding it. In this way we might have fewer emotionally disturbed and psychotic children.

Finally, we feel that the law in relation to cruelty to children should be amended. Legal proceedings may be taken against parents for physical cruelty and the word 'battered baby' is now, unfortunately, commonly used. We have seen many cases of mental cruelty towards children causing severe emotional disturbance. Nothing can be done to remove these children from the disturbing environment, provided there is no physical violence towards them. Unfortunately, many parents are quite unfit to have control of children because of their mental attitude. The law as it stands at present allows them to continue to exert their mentally cruel attitude towards such children.

Some children, can, of course, be sent to Edith Edwards House School, Banstead. This school was established after our units had been in existence for some years, chiefly as a result of our being unable to find suitable placements for many of the children. The school was started under the auspices of the Department of Education and Science with the Invalid Children's Aid Association as managers, has now been in existence for several years and caters for twenty children of both sexes but with males in the majority. Most of the children are psychotic but there is also a leavening of aphasic children. The school is primarily residential with four terms a year but some children are weekly boarders. The children live in groups of four and each group has a 'mother' who looks after the children's out-of-school welfare and a teacher who looks after their education.

There is also a consultant psychiatrist, a part-time psychologist and a speech therapist. Any intercurrent infections are treated by a local general practitioner. The children can go home on holidays and for occasional weekends while an attempt is made at the school to allow them to lead as normal a life as possible—for example, they are taken shopping in the village and to parties by their housemother. They can also play on swings and slides and paddle in a pool provided. There are also television sessions and the children can have their own birthday parties. The school is in the charge of Miss Denny who is the headmistress and who is doing a remarkable job with an extremely difficult group of children. They are receiving what we have already mentioned as 'therapeutic education' and we would like to see more children in such educational establishments.

Probably, and certainly in our present state of knowledge, a psychotic child will always remain a handicapped child in the same way as a deaf or blind child. However, there is a great need for further research into the exact nature of their handicap. Some research into their perceptual difficulties has been begun and is continuing at Belmont. This was initiated by Rees and is very much a team effort. Psychiatrist, teacher, educational psychologist, research psychologist, speech therapist and supervisors all have their part to play, pool their findings and learn from each other. But most important they learn from the children. It would be hopeless to try to teach a completely colour-blind child to differentiate between red and green; similarly, some of these children have perceptual deficits as basic as this defect, while some of them have perceptual weaknesses that can be improved by training. It is obviously very important to differentiate between the two, and this involves long, detailed and careful testing, observation and recording by the whole team. These are children, not guinea pigs, and this work can only be done satisfactorily in a warm, secure home-like environment such as the environment in the Children's Unit. The unnatural surroundings of a hospital ward or large unit introduce complications and certainly retard the children's progress.

Having found the basic deficits, the next step is to help the child to overcome them or to find a way around them.

9—Psychological Assessment of Young Autistic Children

Dr. Agatha H. Bowley, Ph.D.

LEARNING DIFFICULTIES

In work with autistic children the psychologist has two main aims in mind—(1) to make as accurate an assessment of the potential of the child as possible and (2) to ascertain the nature of his special learning difficulties.

There are a number of conditions which make these tasks especially difficult. Firstly, the very nature of his illness means that personal relationships are abnormal and it is by no means easy to gain full and lasting co-operation to enable his response to standardized tests to be accurately measured. Secondly, high distractibility and low frustration tolerance are very characteristic of many of these children, especially if some degree of brain damage is present. Thirdly, some degree of hearing loss may be present and uncorrected, and very frequently there is considerable retardation in language development, either in receptive or expressive language.

The best that one can hope to achieve on a first assessment of the young autistic child is some measurable response to a non-verbal test. The Merrill-Palmer or the Ruth Griffiths Developmental Scale give the truest assessment of non-verbal intelligence on these children under five years of age.

However, the fact that the autistic child shows capacity to solve practical problems at or above his age level is no sure indication of his capacity to respond to formal education. Associated with his immaturity of language is his great difficulty in comprehending symbols and in linking symbols with objects or pictures. The autistic child is slow to express his ideas in drawing or to comprehend printed words as meaningful. He also finds difficulty in grasping simple concepts of number. Moreover, he may be able to make simple associations in a practical situation—that a shoe goes on the foot, a hat on the head, a spoon in the mouth, but fail to grasp this when such objects are presented in a pictorial form as in the Nebraska Test of Learning Aptitude. Similarly, without inner language and a well developed system of codifying he has difficulty in making categories or generalizations; for example, these are all fruits you eat, clothes you wear, things that fly in the air, and so on. The non-communicating autistic child remains much longer than the normal child at the sensori-motor stage of learning, showing good capacity to discriminate shape, size and colour when presented in tri-dimensional form, but very limited comprehension of pictures, spoken or written words.

As language training continues with a skilled teacher, the capacity to understand symbols slowly improves. It becomes possible to assess verbal comprehension on a test such as the English Picture Vocabulary Test and to discover special learning problems by means of the Nebraska Scale which gives a learning age rather than a mental age. Many of these children show poor immediate visual memory and poor retention. They appear unable to hold the image of a colour or a pattern in their minds and have great difficulty on sequencing tests, that is, in recalling a series of shapes presented visually or of digits presented orally. On constructional tests and on matching tests they usually do well but some of them show perceptual impairment and, as

Rimland (1964) has suggested, find it impossible to organize their sensations to make sense of their environment. Such children gain a low score on Progressive Matrices, Wisc Block Designs and Nebraska Block Patterns Tests. On the Marianne Frocstig Tests they gain a poor perception quotient, especially on tests requiring the reproduction of shapes or the understanding of spatial relations.

An assessment of language age can be obtained on the Illinois Test of Psycho-Linguistic Abilities, but with young, autistic children under the age of seven, it is often difficult to gain sufficient response to verbal tests. Much of the Stanford-Binet and the W.I.S.C. is, of course, inappropriate for this reason. They do well on tests requiring the use of gesture to explain function; for example, to show how a telephone or a guitar is used when pictures of these are shown. They may be able to associate pictures, sock with shoe, spoon with cup correctly and achieve visual decoding tests, that is, recognize different types of chairs or coats or shoes as belonging to the same class.

Psychological assessment does attempt to identify the child's particular areas of difficulty in learning and so suggest possible remedial measures. The child must be taught to distinguish similarities and differences, to match and sort objects, to associate those that go together, to begin to classify and gradually to come to some appreciation of the meaning of symbols. Provided he has adequate or corrected hearing, an autistic child can learn to understand, to use and to read words. Accurate assessment of intelligence and satisfactory teaching of these children depend on both emotional and physical factors. It must be possible to achieve a warm relationship with the child, to gain his co-operation and enlist his desire to succeed, and many autistic children remain withdrawn and detached for a considerable time. They shun close contacts and have limited capacity for sustaining good relationships with people. This is often related to poor early mother-child relationships.

But it has proved possible to overcome this withdrawal by providing a secure, affectionate and stimulating environment.

Physical factors are less easy to eliminate. Distractibility, perseveration, echolalia, and perceptual disabilities are very common in children with brain damage and are typical of children with cerebral palsy. Some aphasic children have similar disabilities. The teaching of these children has to be carefully structured and aimed to reinforce and build up links between visual, auditory, tactual and kinaesthetic experiences, providing short periods of concentrated work on a task within their capacity. The more intelligent the child the better the prognosis, for he will be able to invent more compensatory techniques to overcome his disabilities. It is also of great importance to identify these children early and work out remedial techniques in the early stages of learning.

CASE STUDY—(A.C.) A NON-COMMUNICATING CHILD

This little boy first showed symptoms of being withdrawn and non-communicative at the age of two or three years. A study of his early case history showed that he had been six weeks postmature—his mother had also had a prolonged labour at the time of his birth. He had sat up at six months, walked at two years and had full bladder and bowel control by the time he was three and a half. His only attempt at speech had been a little babbling.

Medical findings

Medical findings concluded possible high tone deafness, R-internal strabismus, an abnormal EEG showing possible parietal region damage. An x-ray of his skull, and an analysis of his blood and urine revealed nothing abnormal. His vision and hearing were also normal.

Family circumstances

The boy's father was irritable and suffered from some sexual abnormality. Because the home had been tense and unhappy the parents had divorced and his mother had remarried. The step-father was placid and had a good relationship with the child. By the time this boy had reached the age of four he still had very limited speech. He was hyperactive and distractible and, in addition to this, he was afraid of dogs and open spaces.

Psychological findings

At four years three months (August, 1965) an accurate intellectual assessment was still impossible. He was still hyperactive, and his interests were variable. He showed limited persistence but did have some judgment of shape. At this stage he was judged to be possibly retarded, although by now he could manage some phrases and a few simple words.

At the age of five A.C. was admitted as an inpatient to the Belmont Hospital Children's Unit. His discrimination of shape, size and colour were average and any phrases, sentences or words that were said clearly were carefully noted. His I.Q. was 100 according to the Merrill-Palmer Scale. Two months after admission his word count had reached 20 words but there was no response to the Picture Vocabulary Test, and no concept of numbers. He also failed the Skemp Visual Concepts Tests. In Spatial Relationships he failed the six cube pyramid test. He was still noticeably restless.

At the age of five years five months, A.C. had the learning capacity of a child four and a half, according to the Nebraska Test of Learning Aptitude. His speech was improving but he found tri-dimensional material easier than pictorial material. In play activity he showed some constructive ability and his capacity for concentration was improving. But he did need a transitional object (for example, a shopping bag) to carry around with him. One month later, A.C. was given the Monfraix-Tardieu Perception Test, which showed that he could match factually common objects but not geometrical shapes.

In December, 1966, A.C. had achieved the learning capacity of a child five years of age, although by this time he himself had reached the age of five years seven months. He had also developed a better capacity for concentration. His Vineland Social Age was four years, five months.

In January, 1967 A.C. again failed the Skemp Visual Concepts Test—in Spatial Relationships, manikin four year level. He again failed the six cube pyramid, a test which a normal child of four and a half can pass. As far as number concepts were concerned, he had reached the level of a three year old child.

His language was spontaneous and his speech was quickly developing—nouns, some verbs, phrases and sentences and a few pronouns. He could now indicate pictures when named, and there was no distortion of body image.

Treatment

A.C. was recommended for remedial teaching in a small hospital unit where he was also given speech therapy and operant conditioning.

Summary

During a period of seventeen months this boy has improved considerably in comprehension and use of language, but he remains retarded in conceptual development and apparently in spatial perception. His attention span is limited and some emotional disturbance is evident— his fears and his attachment to certain objects. He is still a difficult child to teach but his social relationships are good. He was finally accepted in a school for maladjusted non-communicating children where he made steady progress. He has been diagnosed as a dysphasic child.

10—Auditory Assessment

Joan E. Taylor, B.A., Diploma of the National College of Teachers of the Deaf

INTRODUCTORY

If we did not depend on excellent hearing for learning and using spoken language as a means of communication we could live quite happily with a severe hearing loss. The primary purpose of auditory assessment is to discover whether the patient's hearing for speech is normal or defective. To test hearing for speech is to test hearing for very quiet sounds. The question to be answered is: "Can this person recognize these words when they are given in a quiet voice at six feet—'sit', 'thick', 'sip', 'fit', 'sick', 'ship'?" If he can his hearing is within normal limits. In effect the question asks whether the patient can hear the difference between 's', 'th', 'f', and 'k', 'p', 't', as used in quiet speech.

A simple, standardized test of hearing, which partly answers the question, uses pure tones from 128 c/s by octaves to 8,192 c/s, a frequency range which covers that of the sounds of speech, to plot a line which shows the decibel level at which the patient says that each tone disappears out of hearing. This line is a useful statement which can be used to compare a person's hearing with a standardized norm.

This line describes what is called the patient's 'threshold

of hearing'. All sounds with a less decibel level cannot be heard; sounds with a greater decibel level, or 'above threshold', can be heard. A person with normal hearing, with a threshold of 0–10 dB, hears sounds of 30 dB as a very quiet whisper. The sounds 'p', 'ch', 's', as used in quiet speech, are to him 40–50 dB. The vowels, 'ar', 'or', as used in ordinary conversation, are to him about 60 dB, but if they are shouted close to his ear they are to him 90 dB.

A person with a 30 dB loss of hearing across the speech range of frequencies has his threshold of hearing at a 30 dB level. If he listens very carefully in a quiet room he can hear the quiet consonants of speech, which sound to him only as loud as 10–20 dB above his threshold of hearing. Voice at 60 dB he hears as a quiet murmur of 30 dB. All speech appears to him quiet and muted.

If this were the only effect of hearing loss, deafness would not be the crippling handicap that it is. A hearing aid would restore the decibel level and all would be well. The other effect of deafness of cochlear origin, and to some degree of conductive deafness, which accompanies loss of loudness, is that similar sounds sound alike. The more severe the hearing loss, the more sounds appear to lose their distinguishing characteristic and approximate to a neutral, unrecognizable sound. A hearing aid does not restore hearing to normal, but merely amplifies the neutral sound. A characteristic response of severely deaf patients is that they are unable to distinguish by hearing alone 'b', 'd', 'g' from a quiet knock on wood; 'p', 't', 'k' from a pencil tap and 's', 'sh', 'f' from the rustle of tissue paper even when these sounds are amplified to a level of 30–40 dB above their threshold of hearing for sounds in this range of frequency.

There are then two principal matters to investigate when making an assessment of hearing. The first is the acuity of the patient's hearing—the decibel level in each ear at which sounds of different frequency are just perceived. The second is how efficiently the patient is able to discriminate between similar sounds. A child who has no words must nevertheless be tested with sounds as quiet as 's', 'th', 'f', the quietest sounds of speech, and his response must show whether he can differentiate between them. That a child notices or responds to a sound merely shows that it is loud enough to him to catch his attention; that is to say, it is at least 20 dB, probably 30–40 dB, above his threshold of hearing. Auditory avoidance or auditory inattention could prevent a child from responding to a sound even though he has acute hearing. A habit of auditory avoidance could prevent him from learning to recognize sounds.

When dealing with a non-communicating child one can say that if he notices a sound, then sounds in that frequency range and of that level of loudness are above his threshold of hearing. If he recognizes the sound he has good hearing in those frequencies. If he understands spoken language, whether he himself speaks or not, he has acute discrimination for quiet sounds across the range of frequencies for speech. If he does not respond to sound one cannot be sure that he does not hear.

An outpatient interview gives one very little time to do a complex job. Time is saved by working systematically and by using tests which give more than one kind of information so that response to one test can be checked against response to another. The tests used here were developed and used during 1957–1966 in the Assessment Centre of the Yorkshire Residential School for the Deaf on 472 children, in addition to the pupils of the school, who were referred for audiologic assessment. The children ranged in age from six months to sixteen years and 317 of them were between two years and seven years. In 1957, individual hearing aids were issued to all pupils in schools for the deaf and records were kept over nine years as a means of assessing the value of hearing aids to children with different degrees of hearing loss. The collected records of the children's responses show how ability to discriminate between similar sounds falls off in proportion as acuity diminishes. The speech audiogram was designed and used as a statement of a child's ability to distinguish speech sounds by hearing alone, and particularly as a way of interpreting the commonly used pure tone audiogram in terms understandable to the parents of the children. The severely deaf and profoundly deaf children who were seen were admitted to the school. Their hearing for speech was periodically assessed throughout their school life. Although the children learned to use their residual hearing to acquire speech by listening to amplified speech combined with speechreading, strict tests of hearing showed that their ability to discriminate between similar sounds did not improve but was a stable condition, although the skilled use of visual clues by the children gave an appearance of improvement.

The hearing of a patient can be investigated by the evaluation of what he has already learned through hearing, and by his response in a test situation. Language is learned in the normal way by hearing it. If a child recognizes words and understands language appropriate to his age level, his hearing is within normal limits. Speech is learned by hearing it, imitating it and matching the imitation by means of auditory feedback. If a small child uses speech sounds correctly in words there is probably little or no significant hearing loss, and tests of hearing in this case would use exceedingly quiet sounds, and especially the sounds of speech. The kind of faults and deviation from normal articulation which appear in the child's own speech as well as articulation skills which could have been acquired only through the use of auditory feedback are indications useful in the assessment of hearing. Other matters which are learned through hearing and which may be observed in the child are the recognition of sounds, association of sound with its source and an ability to locate the source of the sound.

An assessment of hearing can be made from such observed data, but response in a specific test situation is often needed to confirm it. We can know that a person hears a sound only if he tells us or shows us that he does. A disturbed child may hear but be unable or unwilling to show that he hears. The best procedure seems to be to

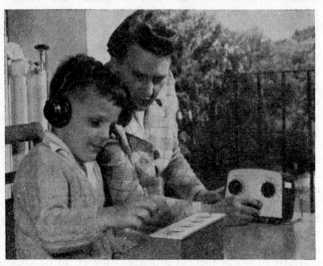

Figure 4. Child having hearing tests.

bear in mind what one wants to know, that is, whether the child hears quiet sounds well enough to be able to tell the difference between 's', 'sh', 'f'; 'p', 't', 'k' as used in quiet speech, and to adapt the method of eliciting a response to the particular child being studied. At the lowest level of performance one can try to get an involuntary response from the child. Sounds of known frequency and monitored level can be made and note taken of whether the child notices, locates, recognizes, imitates, echoes or comments.

Quiet sounds are used. Hearing for speech cannot be tested by using loud sounds. If the child is able to pay attention and co-operate with the examiner he may be persuaded to learn to respond to sounds in simple games by means of which the acuity of his hearing and his ability to distinguish particular sounds may be demonstrated. Some children will be able to give an intelligent response, discussing with the examiner what they hear, or if they have no language, indicating whether the testing sounds are heard or not, in right or left ear, how loud they appear to be and perhaps say whether they are high or low tones.

The assessment begins as soon as the child arrives for the interview. The child's conduct and personality are observed, his relationship with his mother and the mother's management of the child. Throughout the interview the examiner continually evaluates what the child has which he could only have learned through hearing; attention to environmental sounds, familiar voices, footsteps, trains passing, crockery, music, tones of voice, laughing, crying, sounds outside the room; location of the source of sound, recognition of sound, association with source, association with meaning; understanding spoken language; use of speech.

CASES QUOTED

Seven cases are used to illustrate the points made.

(1) E.R. was a girl of 6 years, 5 months whose language was retarded and who had a speech defect.

(2) L.L. was a boy of 8 years, 3 months who had a severe speech defect and very much retarded language.

(3) P.W. was a boy of 5 years, 9 months whose speech was almost unintelligible and who understood only very simple language.

These children were seen as outpatients and their cases illustrate the effects of hearing loss in otherwise normal children.

(4) N.N. was a boy of 7 years, 7 months who had been a short term inpatient during his fifth year, and was seen again as an outpatient. His language had developed but he still had very faulty speech. His case notes are quoted to illustrate the difference between speech faults caused by deafness and those caused by structural abnormality.

(5) E.E., a girl of 6 years, 9 months, was seen first as an outpatient, but was then admitted as an inpatient for three weeks for a more complete study to be made. Her notes show the difference between the response of a severely subnormal child and a profoundly deaf child to auditory stimuli.

(6) Y.T. was a little girl of 7 years, 10 months with a possible hearing loss underlying a personality disorder. She was first seen as an outpatient and then for a month as an inpatient. Her case is quoted as it shows some of the difficulties met with when dealing with a disturbed child.

(7) L.S. was admitted at 5 years, 2 months as an inpatient and stayed for a year. He was a boy of above average intelligence who had a severe receptive dysphasia. His case was interesting on account of the shifts and dodges and *ad hoc* tests which were devised to wake in him some response to auditory stimuli. He had to be taught to listen before he could be tested. We had to know whether he was totally deaf, deaf and dysphasic, or whether he had a severe receptive dysphasia but no hearing loss.

These children were seen as inpatients. Their cases are described in detail in this chapter.

CASE 1—E.R.

Female outpatient with an I.Q. of 100 and a learning age of six years, six months; actual age was six years, five months.

Aetiology—Intermittent conductive deafness in infancy and early childhood; auditory inattention; still minor partial deafness (HOH) particularly in high tones; no structural abnormalities.

Early history—No understandable words until after three years; no sentences until after four years, six months.

Personality and conduct—Rather shy; self-contained; obedient good co-operation.

E.R. 6 years 5 months

Sounds used for Freefield tests

	Low	Middle	High frequencies
	Drum tapped with fingers Quiet knock	Quiet rattle Bell 2 pencils gently knocked Bead in little toy cupboard	Quiet bell Whistle Chime bar 4000 c/s Drum stroked with fingers Tissue paper
Level of sound	30-40 dB	40 dB	40-50 dB
Approximate threshold	10-20 dB	20 dB	20-30 dB

Figure 5. These sounds, made as quietly as possible, were loud enough to attract her attention. They were therefore at least 20 dB above her threshold of hearing.

Tests of hearing

Two acuity tests of hearing were given to E.R. during an interview as an outpatient.

(1) *Freefield test*—E.R. was first given some little dolls and dolls' furniture to play with while her mother was talking. Quiet sounds were made behind her, out of her field of vision; for example, something rattling inside a little toy cupboard. When E.R. turned to see what it was, she was given the toy. She noticed rattles, small bells and quiet whistles. All these sounds were as quiet as they could be

made. E.R. responded to these sounds as though she heard them quiet well. They were not so near her threshold of hearing that she had to listen very carefully for them but were at least 20 dB above threshold. She located these sounds given behind on the left and behind on the right. Her response to this test gave a baseline from which to work.

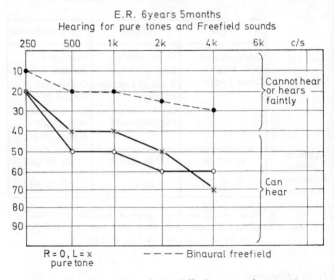

Figure 6. Young children find it difficult to attend to meaningless sounds close to their threshold of hearing. The sounds (pure tone) here recorded are probably 15–20 dB above threshold.

(2) *Pure tone audiometer test*—During the preliminary interview and the Freefield test, E.R. showed that she could both understand and use simple language and that she was friendly and able to co-operate in a test with the pure tone audiometer. She put the headphones on and was shown

116

that different sounds could be made loud or quiet and put into either ear. She was asked to respond by saying whether the sound was there or not, which ear it was in, and how loud it was.

Her actual response was recorded, but young, disturbed children find it difficult to attend to sounds close to the threshold of hearing and the sounds recorded are probably at least 15–20 dB above threshold.

These two tests of acuity of hearing show which frequencies of hearing are perceived at which levels of loudness. It was not thought necessary to ask E.R. to do a test to show that she could discriminate between similar sounds. She had demonstrated that she could do this by learning to speak.

The next tests E.R. was given were the Speech Tests of Hearing. A cochlear hearing loss is two dimensional: (1) sounds appear fainter (2) similar sounds sound alike. If E.R.'s pure tone audiogram is reliable, and if her hearing loss is a peripheral loss, *Figure 7*, which shows speech sounds related to the pure tone audiogram, will also show what difficulties E.R. might be expected to have when listening to speech.

Five simple speech tests of hearing were next given to E.R.

(1) *Numbers one to ten*—E.R. was given a card on which the numbers 1–10 were randomly placed. She listened without watching the speaker's face. The numbers were named in a quiet voice two feet away. E.R. pointed to the numerals named.

She had no difficulty in recognizing the numbers 1–6 because each has a different vowel and her hearing for vowels was good. She gave a hesitant, slow response whenever 7, 8, 9 and 10 were used, but did get them right. She was more quick and sure with clearer, closer speech.

(2) *Belmont Speech Hearing Test*—The Belmont Speech Hearing Test uses a card on which fifteen pictures and the

117

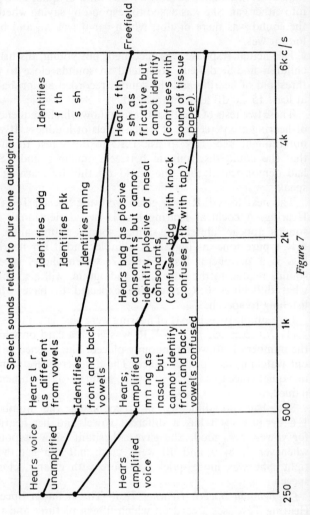

E.R. 6 years 5 months

Speech sounds related to pure tone audiogram

Hears voice unamplified	Hears l r as different from vowels	Identifies bdg Identifies ptk	Identifies f th s sh
	Identifies front and back vowels	Identifies mnng	
Hears; amplified voice	Hears; amplified mn ng as nasal but cannot identify front and back vowels confused	Hears bdg as plosive consonants but cannot identify plosive or nasal consonants (confuses bdg with knock confuses ptk with tap).	Hears f th s sh as fricative but cannot identify (confuses with sound of tissue paper).

250   500   1k   2k   4k   6kc/s

Freefield

Figure 7

118

numerals 1–6 are drawn. Good hearing for consonants is required to obtain a full score.

tree	1	shoe	knife	cap	4	fish
house	5	cow	fork	ship	2	face
scissors	3	cat	spoon	door	6	hat

The above words were given in a different order in a quiet voice at two feet. E.R. listened without watching the speaker's face and pointed to the picture named. She confused

tree/three	two/shoe/spoon	four/fork

When the words were given no louder, but with clearer, more deliberate speech, she made no mistake.

(3) *Repeat Speech Sounds*—Twenty speech sounds were given in a quiet voice at two feet on the right. E.R. was required to listen (without watching) and to say what she heard each time. She was not corrected. What she did say was noted.

ba	oo	m	sh	t	or	da	n	s	ee
p	ga	k	la	f	ar	th	oh	ch	ja

E.R. heard them all. She confused

m/n	ga/ba	k/t	s/sh	f/th

The sounds were given no louder, but at one foot on the left. E.R. made no mistake.

In normal life one is not often required to deal with single sounds and words, but with polysyllabic words and phrases which are more easily recognized because they offer more clues.

(4) *Ten disyllabic words*—When ten disyllabic words were given in clear, close, quiet speech, E.R. made no mistake. The toys named were present and their names were familiar; this helped to give her some clues.

(5) *Repeat Common Phrases*—E.R. had no difficulty with

these. The results of the Speech Tests of Hearing are summarized in *Figure 8*.

Understanding and use of spoken language

E.R. understood ordinary conversation except some remarks which had to be repeated in clear, deliberate speech

E.R. 6years 5months
Summary of results of speech tests of hearing

SPEECH AUDIOGRAM		
Amplification R:nil L:nil quiet speech 2 ft on Rt	Recognizes type of sound	Identifies individual sounds
Voice	Hears voice unamplified	
Vowels	✓	✓
Continuants	✓	✓
Nasal consonants	✓	m n confused
Voiced plosives	✓	g b confused
Breathed plosives	✓	k t confused
Fricatives	✓	f th s sh confused

Figure 8. On left: with clearer articulation she made no mistakes.

while she was watching and some remarks had to be rephrased in simpler language as for a child much younger than six years, six months.

E.R. talked readily but the language she used was immature. It sounded like the language of a normal child, but a younger, normal child. She had some faults in

120

articulation of a kind fairly common in a younger child's speech—'sh' for 's'; 'd' for 'th'; 't' for 's'.

There was a neatness about her articulation which belonged to speech learned naturally—by hearing it, and using auditory feedback to correct it. In the sentence 'What do you want' the 't' of 'what' was held and correctly exploded as 'd'. The 't' of 'want' was exactly right. For 'sixpence' she said 'tikpent' but the 'k' was held and exploded as 'p'.

These refinements of articulation are learned by hearing them and monitoring one's own speech by auditory feedback.

E.R.'s response to all tests of hearing shows good hearing for low sounds, and a slight loss of hearing for sounds of middle and high frequency. This has not been severe enough to have prevented her from learning spoken language in the normal way. It could however, have caused frequent uncertainty which would perhaps account for the general immaturity of her spoken language.

As a baby and as a small child E.R. would have been spoken to at close range with much repetition. These are precisely the conditions which a slight hearing loss demands. As she has grown older she has had to deal with sound from a distance and in noisier surroundings. Consequently, her handicap began to show effect. Her best help would probably be a habit of speechreading. If she still has periodic conductive deafness, a bone conduction hearing aid could be provided for her to wear at her own discretion.

CASE 2—L.L.

Male outpatient with an I.Q. of 92 and a learning capacity described as 'low average'. His age was eight years, three months.

Aetiology—M.Rh. negative; jaundiced; exchange transfusion after five days; early diagnosis as receptive dysphasic; there were no structural abnormalities.

Early history—Severe speech defect and very retarded language; jaundice requiring exchange transfusion after five days showed risk of other damage in addition to cochlear deafness.

Personality and conduct—Friendly; worked well and cheerfully at the tests he was given.

Test of hearing

The pure tone audiometer test was given to L.L. during an interview. He, too, was an outpatient.

Pure tone audiogram—L.L. willingly wore the headphones of the pure tone audiometer. He had had previous experience of these, but was shown again that sounds of different pitch could be made loud or quiet in either ear. He responded by saying in which ear the sound was, how loud it was and when it was no longer there. L.L.'s pure tone audiogram showed a severe hearing loss in the middle frequencies of the speech range.

	250	500	1,000	2,000	4,000	6,000	c/s
				L.L.'s pure tone audiogram			
Right ear	30	30	55	70	70	55	dB
Left ear	15	30	35	70	45	40	dB

The audiogram of an eight year old boy who co-operates fully and intelligently in the test is probably within 5–10 dB of his threshold of hearing.

Middle frequency loss

If these scores are averaged, L.L. would appear to have not much worse a loss than E.R., the previous case described, but whereas her loss was in the high frequencies, L.L.'s loss was in the middle frequencies. This has proved to be the more crippling loss.

In *Figure 9* L.L.'s audiogram is related to the sounds of speech and shows that if his audiogram is accurate and his deafness is of cochlear origin, one would expect him to

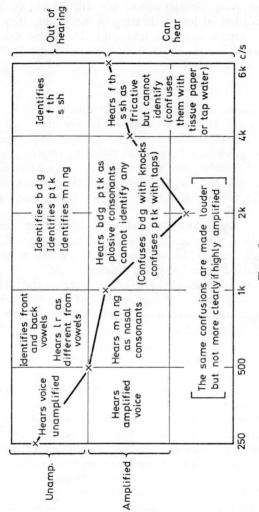

L.L. 8 years 3 months

Speech sounds related to pure tone audiogram

	250	500	1k	2k	4k	6k c/s

Unamp.
Hears voice unamplified

Amplified

Identifies front and back vowels
Hears l r as different from vowels

Hears m n ng as nasal consonants

Hears amplified voice

Identifies b d g
Identifies p t k
Identifies m n ng

Hears b d g p t k as plosive consonants cannot identify any
(Confuses b d g with knocks confuses p t k with taps)

Identifies f th s sh

Hears f th s sh as fricative but cannot identify (confuses them with tissue paper or tap water)

Out of hearing

Can hear

[The same confusions are made louder but not more clearly if highly amplified]

Figure 9

have poor discrimination for all speech sounds. The indication of loss of hearing in the middle frequencies is that similar sounds sound alike. The worse the loss, the more all sounds are levelled to one indistinguishable buzz.

Speech tests of hearing

Speech tests of hearing confirmed that L.L. had this difficulty. He heard unamplified voice quite well but confused front and back vowels. The five simple speech tests were given to L.L., with the following results.

(1) *Numbers one to ten*—L.L. confused two/three and one/nine, and was uncertain about all the other numbers.

(2) *Belmont Speech Hearing Test*—No reliable score was obtained.

(3) *Repeat Speech Sounds*—L.L. heard all the sounds, but could not distinguish between similar sounds: 's', 'sh' and 'f' all sounded like 'sh'. Similarly, 'd', 'b' and 'g' all sounded alike and he had to guess which was said.

(4) *Ten disyllabic words*—Toys were on the table to give him some clue and each word had its own characteristic shape, which gave some small clue. Out of the ten, four were scored right.

> basket   rabbit   scissors   tractor   lorry
> teapot   sixpence   motor   pencil   hammer

(5) *Repeat Common Phrases*—L.L. recognized the familiar outlines of seven out of 25 without speechreading. When allowed to speechread, he got all of them right.

This is a typical performance of a child with a severe perceptual hearing loss. His response to sound was consistent. Whether the sounds are pure tones or speech sounds, he responds to the same frequency band consistently. This would seem to rule out receptive dysphasia as a diagnosis.

L.L. has taught himself to speechread, to supplement his faulty hearing by watching speakers' faces. Through this he has a fairly good understanding of simple language.

Very familiar words and phrases he 'hears' quite well if
there are situational clues to help to give meaning, but new
words and new turns of speech he needs to speechread.
Speechreading is not a wholly reliable means of communication, so he is constantly on the edge of error in understanding
what people are saying to him.

L.L. 8years 3 months
Summary of results of speech tests of hearing

SPEECH AUDIOGRAM		
Amplification R:nil L:nil	Recognizes type of sound	Identifies individual sound
Voice	Hears voice unamplified	
Vowels	✓	Confuses front + back vowels
Continuants	R + L confused with vowels	
Nasal consonants	hears as nasal	No recognition of any sound by hearing alone
Voiced plosives	hears as plosives	
Breathed plosives	hears as bd plosives	
Fricatives	hears as fricative	

*Figure 10. L.L. relies on speechreading for recognition of all
speech sounds because of severe deafness.*

His language is retarded in that he suffers from the
deprivation usual to deaf people, is unable to overhear
general conversation and has to manage with only such
communication as is made directly to him face to face.
His speech is intelligible in the main. It is an echo of what
is poorly heard. He has poor auditory feedback of his own
speech and cannot use this to correct his articulation.

A hearing aid would help L.L. to hear the high fricative

consonants, but with vowel hearing at 15 dB he would not be able to tolerate enough amplification to make the middle frequency sounds available.

L.L. needs much help with language. The better his understanding of language, the better he will appear to hear.

CASE 3—P.W.

Male outpatient with an I.Q. of 100, aged five years, nine months.

Aetiology—Congenital total peripheral deafness; retarded language and very poor speech; tongue-tie operation at four years.

Early history—Hearing aids and peripatetic help from one year; school for the deaf at two years.

Personality and conduct—Friendly; good co-operation; used to working with adults.

P.W. was a friendly little boy, very ready to do what he was asked. The following assessment was carried out during an outpatient interview.

Tests of hearing

P.W. was given two tests of acuity of hearing.

(1) *Freefield test*—The only sound P.W. heard was a large drum struck close behind him.

(2) *Pure tone audiometer test*—P.W. gave no response to the pure tone audiometer which amplified low frequency sounds to a level at which he could hear them. He did not respond to the chime bars (500–4,000 c/s) but did hear voice ('go') amplified through the speech training amplifier at 95 dB.

As far as discrimination was concerned, P.W. showed no useful hearing for speech even when words were spoken into two hearing aids. *Figure 11* summarizes the effect of profound hearing loss on hearing for speech.

P.W. 5 years 9 months
Hearing for speech. Summary of test results

Speech audiogram		
Amplification R:95, L 95 dB	Recognizes type of sound	Identifies sound
Voice	Aware of voice highly amplified no discrimination	
Vowels		
Continuants		
Nasal consonants		
Voiced plosives	No response	
Breathed plosives		
Fricatives		

Figure 11. P.W. relies on speechreading for all receptive language. He is totally deaf to speech and profoundly deaf to all sound.

Spoken language

Understanding and use—P.W. understood very simple language through reading and speechreading.

Speech—P.W. used his voice very readily and his approximate speech projectively to communicate ideas. His speech is almost unintelligible because of poor tongue control. If one had a clue to what he was saying and listened very carefully, one could make out what he was saying, provided one also watched his mouth, to get a hint by speechreading.

A normally hearing child who had a tongue-tie operated at four years might still have some speech faults a year later. A profoundly deaf boy would, of course, have more difficulty. He has to develop control for speech through the feedback of his teacher's approval. That he has succeeded to

127

the extent that he has would seem to show a child with no other severe defect than his peripheral deafness.

CASE 4—N.N.

Male outpatient with an I.Q. of 117 (W.I.S.C. 86) aged seven years, one month.

Aetiology—Multiple congenital abnormalities; congenital short palate; palsy; speech faulty.

Early history—Severe executive dysphasia; at four years, two months he attended the children's unit as a daily out-patient for one month.

Personality and conduct—Formerly withdrawn; negativistic response.

N.N. was a friendly little boy who worked well at the tests with good co-operation and attention.

He showed no loss on the pure tone audiometer test, nor on any speech tests of hearing. He used normal language freely and naturally, talked about his play and held conversation. He heard well enough to perceive the difference between his own articulation and that of a person correcting him and trying to improve his speech.

N.N.'s chief difficulty was in the articulation of consonants. His vowels were approximately correct but were lax and nasal. Most of his consonants were faulty.

Plosive consonants

'b' is recognizable, but sounds rather like 'mb'. 'd', 'g', have nasal escape of air: (nɔ) door, (n͡gi͡ŋ) digging 'p', 't'. He can pronounce these fairly well singly, but in words they approximate to (m) or (n) or in some positions in a word a glottal stop°is used. °

　　　　(ɸmuːn) spoon,　　(xɑ') cat,　　(xɑm) cap.

For 't', 'k', he̊ used a velar fricative sound°(like (x) in Scottish loch)　　(xʎ̃ʔ) tree,　　(xʎɑ̃ʰn̥ɑ̃) tractor.

128

Fricative consonants

'f' is faint but recognizable.

For other fricative sounds (ʃ, s, θ.) and the affricate ch, (tʃ) he used the sounds written here as (ʄ).

This sound he made not by using his tongue, but by clenching his teeth, tensing the sides of his mouth and making a fricative sound like that of a small child playing trains.

N.N. was able to control his soft palate well enough to produce the strongly fricative sound (ʄ) and also the unvoiced velar fricative (x), and the voiced velar fricative (g), in (nˀgĩŋ), digging.

N.N. has poor control of the blade of his tongue and has difficulty with 's', 'sh', 'r', 'ch', 't', 'n', 'l'. An additional proof that N.N. hears well is that he makes a difference between 'three' which he calls (ʄʎiː) and 'tree', which he pronounces as (xʎiː). Similarly, he distinguishes between 'cat' (xɑˀ), and 'cap' (xɑm̥).

The kind of speech faults which a child develops are some clue to his difficulty.

N.N., a dysarthric child, is able to invent pronunciations for himself which he substitutes for the speech sounds he is unable to master. He uses his own auditory feedback to match these sounds as near as he can to the correct sounds. This can be done only by a person who has very good hearing.

A child with a partial hearing loss has not only poor hearing for another person's speech, but also poor auditory feedback for his own. His own auditory feedback tells him that he has matched what he has heard fairly well, and it must be difficult for him to understand why other people say his speech is incorrect.

A totally deaf child has no auditory feedback. He has to match kinaesthetically what he perceives visually. His faults are that he substitutes other lip, tongue and mouth movements which look like the ones he perceives; 'm' for 'b', 'l' for 'n' or 't', and omits the ones he does not see.

The speech of a dyspraxic child has an overall laxness, as though he is muttering under his breath.

CASE 5—E.E.

Female inpatient with an I.Q. of 32; learning age two years, three months; actual age six years, nine months.

Aetiology—Severely subnormal intelligence on the basis of brain damage; inattentive to sound when visually engaged.

Early history—Variously diagnosed from one year as deaf, ineducable, psychotic; at three years she was admitted to a day nursery but was excluded because of anti-social behaviour; admitted to a training centre at four years but was removed by mother after one week.

Personality and conduct—No speech; with an I.Q. of 32 showed the conduct disorders of the severely subnormal; could co-operate only in simple mechanical activities; attention span of two to three minutes at the utmost. E.E. was a little girl who was a short-term inpatient. The following observations were made during her stay.

Play when not directed

E.E. scrambled about after large, round beads which she had scattered on the floor, knocking them about and laughing. She enjoyed swinging things and throwing them and emptying boxes. E.E. also undressed a doll and licked it all over. She handled a rubber quoit and a ball; she licked them all over but would not play with them.

E.E. played with a rolling rattle and a plastic egg which contained shot, chuckling and laughing at the movement and perhaps the sound. She fumbled with a formboard until some of the pieces went in. She could not put nesting

CASES QUOTED

E.E 6years 9months

Freefield audiogram

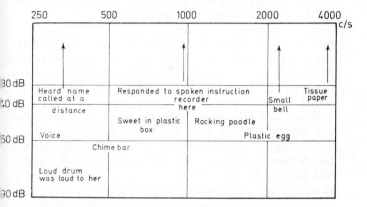

Figure 12. All these sounds were loud enough to take her attention and therefore 20–30 dB above her threshold of hearing.

boxes together but could thread beads and usually did three or four before she gave up.

A nursery rhyme record was put on. E.E. did not look at it but rolled on her back on the floor with knees and elbows bent, smiling and chuckling like a small baby.

Response to sound

E.E. was fairly biddable in a controlled situation. She had the uninhibited conduct of the severely subnormal. It was not useful to give her the usual battery of tests of hearing. It seemed that better results would be obtained by careful observation of her behaviour over a period of time with simple *ad hoc* tests of hearing whenever she could be induced to give her attention.

E.E. was placed at a table with a pegboard and large pegs and was helped to put in one peg each time a drum was

131

struck in front of her. She blinked at the sound as though it was loud. She was shown 14 times before she put in a peg without being prompted. She then put a peg in every time the drum struck behind her, seven times.

Next day, after 10 showings, E.E. would put pegs in to a moderately loud drum struck behind her. After six showings she put pegs in when the 500 c/s chime bar was struck behind her. She smiled when she first heard this and looked round to see what it was, recognizing that it was a different sound.

Afterwards E.E. played with the chime bars for about two minutes, striking them, listening and laughing.

Next day E.E. noticed the sound of a kelly poodle (music chime when it rocks [middle frequencies] 40–50 dB). She played with this for about three minutes, knocking it, running away and coming back to it. E.E. was given some small bricks to play with on a felt covered tray. She moved them around and piled up two or three. She very soon lost interest and as soon as she did, a sweet which had been wrapped in tissue paper was gently unwrapped behind her. She turned to this very quiet sound and was given the sweet. Later, when she was engaged with a simple shapes form-board, the same sound was made again. She ignored it this time.

Next day E.E. was placed at a table with a quiet mechanical occupation, putting pegs into holes. A small plastic box with a sweet in it was rattled near her. She took no notice—still no notice when it came within peripheral vision, nor when it touched her hair. When it came right in front she took it, opened it and ate the sweet. This happened six times, at intervals. The seventh and eighth time E.E. turned to the box when it was rattled behind her. (The sound was low middle frequencies about 40–50 dB.)

This game has been played with her many times in various places; going downstairs, in the dining room, in the kitchen. Often she noticed it. Several times she ignored it. She is very fond of sweets but did not seem able to associate the rattle of the box which she heard with the concept of sweets inside it.

Other quiet freefield sounds which she has heard and located are: a recorder note (1,000 c/s), tissue paper (4–5,000 c/s), a very small bell (c. 3,000 c/s) and a small rattle (c. 1–2,000 c/s). She located the small rattle when it was sounded under the table and also enjoyed hearing and playing the xylophone.

E.E. would react to a sharp command, when she did not see the speaker's face. When she was called by name from the corridor, E.E., who was in the office, ran out. This, of course, proved that she recognized her own name. She also obeyed many simple commands spoken when she was not watching, such as 'put your shoes on', 'bring me your socks', 'give me the soap', 'come and sit down'. E.E. had no words. She hummed with a pleasant, normal-sounding tone and also giggled and laughed. Sounds which had evoked response on several occasions were placed on an audiogram form and seemed to indicate that E.E. had no hearing loss which could have prevented speech from developing in the normal way.

CASE 6—Y.T.

Female inpatient (short-term, one month) with an I.Q. of 86 but with some scores average; seven years, ten months old.

Aetiology—Premature; paranatal brain damage of prematurely born infant; neuro-developmental disorder, maximum defect being in the reception and execution of speech; receptive dysphasia over and above hearing loss.

Early history—Only child in a household of adults; period in a school for partially hearing (excluded); 50–100 words used as word labels; echoic utterances; no real evidence of breakthrough of language proper; no structural abnormality of speech organs.

133

Personality and conduct—Emotionally labile; negativistic; manipulates people by quick mood change; highly distractible; poor persistance.

Y.T. was a negativistic, emotionally labile, highly distractible child with poor perseverence, who continually manipulated people by quick mood change. She was able to work through the battery of tests of hearing during the month she was resident here.

She was perfectly able to do everything she was asked to do during the tests, but it was necessary first to establish a relationship with her which would result in her giving reliable responses. She could be friendly and co-operative and would work quite hard for ten minutes or so. She would then dissolve into a small, spoilt child crying for mother with real tears. If one waited kindly for a little while, and let her know that this was not real distress, she would dry her eyes, laugh at herself and get to work again or she would take the line that it was real. One then had to be quite firm and let her know that if it was real she must go back to the playroom until she was better. For variation, she would pretend that it was very funny if she just did nothing she was asked to do. The answer to this seemed to be to ignore her completely, and to get on with one's own work. She would then cry for mother, watching carefully for the effect, then sit up straight and say she was ready to work.

Tests of hearing

Acuity test for sound—It was obvious that Y.T. heard voice unamplified, so this was used to establish that she could manage a simple test. She wore the headphones of the speech training amplifier and put out a counter each time she heard the word 'go'. She did this reliably.

The same game was played with her using minimal 's'. This she heard in her left ear at 90 dB, but response on the right was not reliable—she seemed to be guessing. At this level of 90 dB she heard 's' quite well enough to recognize it

134

CASES QUOTED

Y.T. 7years 10months

Speech sounds related to pure tone audiogram

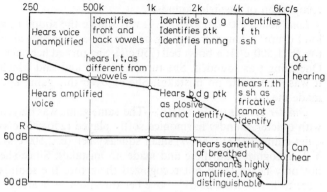

Figure 13

as a fricative sound and to try to indicate it variously, as 'sh' or 'ee' or a high squeak. This is a common, recognized response of a severely deaf child to a high frequency sound.

A test using the chime bars obtained a reliable response; moderately quiet for low sounds, moderately loud for high sounds.

500	1,000	2,000	4,000 c/s.
mp	mp	mf	mf

Pure tone audiogram—In a monaural test using headphones, Y.T. responded to the sounds given to her by saying in which ear she heard them, and whether the sound was there or not. She enjoyed doing this and worked well for short periods. It took several days of checking and rechecking to obtain what seemed to be a reliable score. In *Figure 13* her pure tone audiogram is associated with hearing for speech sounds.

Discrimination

Discrimination of sound involved binaural listening and recognition of freefield sounds.

Loud sound (90–100 dB)—Y.T. was shown the sound of a loud drum; a hammer rapping on a table; a large squeaker toy (c. 1,500 c/s); a brass bell (750 c/s). She turned her back. One thing was sounded. She turned around and said which it was. She made no mistakes. She enjoyed this game and made me do it.

Quieter sounds (c. 50–60 dB)—The same game was played with quieter sounds: harmonica softly played (250–500 c/s) quiet chime bar (1,000 c/s) small squeaky bell (c. 2,500 c/s). Y.T. recognized all these and made no mistakes. Since she not only heard them but recognized them too, the sounds were to her at least 20 dB above her threshold of hearing.

In *Figure 14* the freefield sounds which Y.T. recognized are 'placed' on an audiogram.

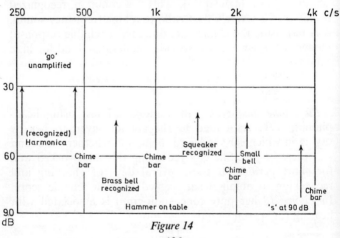

Y.T. 7 years 10 months
Freefield sounds placed on audiogram

Figure 14

136

Hearing for speech

Y.T. was familiar with all the material used in the tests. She could name all the pictures in fairly clear, but faulty, speech. She had between 50 and 100 words which she could use in this way. The phrases used were some which she herself used in ordinary situations. She could also count to ten.

The speech tests of hearing were given several times on different days. The tests were given thus.

(1) Amplified, with speechreading (R.90, L.90 dB).
(2) Unamplified, with speechreading.
(3) Amplified, without speechreading (R. 90, L. 90 dB).
(4) Unamplified, listening alone without speechreading.

Response (c.d.)—If she listened without speechreading, whether with amplification or not, she made no score.

Response (a.b.)—If she speechread and listened, whether the speech was amplified or not, she made no mistakes.

Her response was inconsistent in that she made different errors on different days, and did not even always recognize words which she herself used. Her response was consistent in that she confused words which looked alike.

Four simple speech tests were given to Y.T. with the following results.

(1) Numbers one to ten—Y.T. made no score on the recognition of numbers. She counted to ten, but this was meaningless.

(2) Belmont Speech Hearing Test—Y.T. confused shoe/two, four/fork, house/cow, cat/hat.

(3) Repeat Speech Sounds—Without speechreading she imitated different vowels, but said 'm' sounded like 'bee'; she could not recognize any consonants. With speechreading, she imitated correctly the visible consonants, and could distinguish between b/p, d/t when watching and listening. The consonants, which give poor visual clues ('k', 'g', 'ng'; 's', 'sh', 'ch', 'r') she guessed at and could not reproduce.

Y.T. 7 years 10 months

Summary of speech tests of hearing

SPEECH AUDIOGRAM		
Amplification R: 95 L . 80	Recognizes type of sound	Identifies sound
Voice	Hears voice unamplified	
Vowels	✓	✓
Continuants	✓	Recognizes l
Nasal consonants	Confuses m with front vowel	Confuses m n ng
Voiced plosive ..	✓	Confuses b d g
Breathed plosive ..	Hears something	Confuses all
Fricative consonants	When amplified	Unvoiced consonants

Figure 15

Severely deaf children commonly find articulation of half-seen sounds difficult. They have no auditory feedback by which to correct their speech.

(*4*) *Trisyllabic words and common phrases*—With speech-reading and listening, Y.T. made a better score. She recognized such words as 'teddy-bear', 'pussy-cat', 'motor car' and 'aeroplane'; she confused 'elephant', 'telephone', and also confused 'what is that' with 'pussy-cat'.

In real life situations which gave clues to the meaning of what was said she understood many simple phrases and instructions by speechreading, but was always on the edge of error.

She understood communication by gesture and used mime and gesture herself in a very lively way. She would be lost without it. She used many little spoken phrases; for

138

example, 'never mind', 'wait a minute', 'you do it', 'come in' and 'no, thank you'. As she played she used a great deal of unintelligible babble, with normal sounding intonation, so that at a distance all the vowels appeared and the labial consonants, and 't', 'd', but no fricative sounds or velar consonants. She had no grammar. She could not pivot with words and could not use verbs or prepositions.

Other activities in the classroom showed that she had learning difficulties over and above the effects of hearing loss.

CASE 7—L.S.

Male inpatient with an I.Q. of 121, admitted at the age of five years, two months.

Aetiology—A rubella baby; receptive dysphasia.

Early history—Could not develop any language at all and was referred so that evidence could be established as to whether this was due to a hearing loss, a receptive dysphasia or a severe hearing loss combined with the dysphasia.

Personality and conduct—A pleasant, busy little boy who enjoyed learning.

L.S. was admitted as an inpatient aged about 5 years and stayed in the unit for just over a year. The cause of his disabilities is thought to be his mother's rubella in early pregnancy. L.S. is very fond of his parents who are most concerned for his welfare. Although he had a severe receptive aphasia which prevented him from responding to speech or even to any sound he had some inner system of thinking without words which enabled him to solve problems and manage situations in a way similar to that of a deaf child.

In spite of an additional visuo-perceptual disability which makes it difficult for him to judge spatial relationships he scored an I.Q. of 121. In everything except his failure to respond to sound he is a fun-loving, quick-minded child who enjoys learning.

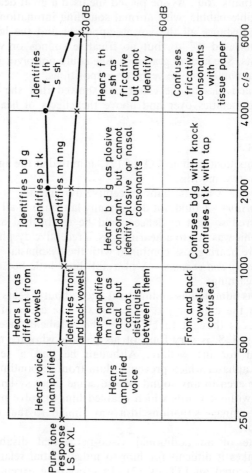

Figure 16. L.S.'s response to pure tone tests and to freefield tests shows that the acuity of his hearing is good enough for him to have learned to understand language and to have developed speech in the normal way. When he has learned to use his hearing to respond to spoken language, he can be given speech tests of hearing which will show whether he has any slight loss in the high frequencies.

The table within the figure reads:

L.S. 5 years 6 months

Speech sounds related to pure tone audiogram

250	500	1000	2000	4000	6000 c/s
Hears voice unamplified	Hears l r as different from vowels		Identifies b d g Identifies p t k	Identifies f th s sh	30 dB
		Identifies front and back vowels	Identifies m n ng		
Hears amplified voice	Hears amplified m n ng as nasal but cannot distinguish between them		Hears b d g as plosive consonant but cannot identify plosive or nasal consonants	Hears f th s sh as fricative but cannot identify	
	Front and back vowels confused		Confuses b d g with knock confuses p t k with tap	Confuses fricative consonants with tissue paper	60 dB

Pure tone response LS or XL

140

In addition to this we soon discovered a great personal self-regard which would not let him make a fool of himself. He was very agile and enjoyed appreciative audiences. He often organized the play of the other children.

The work with him consisted of the following.

(1) Making careful notes of every spontaneous response to sound, and of his own experimenting with sound.

(2) Training him to pay attention to sound, especially to vocal sound and speech.

(3) Making periodic assessment of his hearing using simple tests of various kinds.

The following is a summary of L.S.'s progress, recorded month-by-month, during his one year's stay as an inpatient.

March (250–1,000 c/s at 70–80 dB)

L.S. had many experiments with sound and soon showed interest in sound-making toys. He played musical instruments—glockenspiel (250–500 c/s) harmonica (250–500 c/s) melodica (250–1,000 c/s) for ten or fifteen minutes at a time, playing the different notes, banging in rhythm and rocking to it.

April (250–1,000 c/s at 70–80 dB)

L.S. made no response to audiometers and no response to the 'go' test. He did not appear to locate sounds. There was, however, an indication of spontaneous response; a night nurse reported that when she was dressing L.S. upstairs, a member of staff began to laugh with another child downstairs. L.S. indicated that someone was laughing downstairs. He heard, recognized and located the sound.

May (250–4,000 c/s at 50–70 dB)

L.S. played with every musical instrument and sound-making toy he could find, pretending to sing. The enjoyment and interested attention which he gave to this was the first real evidence that he was by no means totally deaf. He went down to the supervisors and told them what he had been doing.

Pure tone audiogram—During binaural listening using Peter's freefield audiometer, L.S. responded by putting pegs into holes when he heard a sound.

	250	500	1k	2k	4k	c/s
Right and left ear	15	20	20	30	30	

He responded more quickly to sounds of low and low middle frequencies than to those of light middle and high frequencies.

June (*250–4,000 c/s at 50–70 dB*)

In a game suggested by Rees, L.S. was given an electric torch which shone with a red light. A sound was given which he was known to hear well. He was shown that when the sound was made he was to shine the torch on his face. He did not see the movement which caused the sound which was of three or four seconds duration. When he had responded to the sound several times, he was suddenly given a succession of very short sounds. He smiled and immediately responded with many short flashes of the torch. When a high frequency sound was substituted for a low note he seemed to be put out and did not respond. He has shown since that he actually does hear this high note (4,000 c/s).

L.S. was required to put a peg into a board every time he heard the word 'go'. Most children find this one of the easier tasks but L.S. would not respond to the human voice, although he had shown that he heard sounds in this frequency range at the same level (200–500 c/s at 65 dB).

L.S. would not at first wear the headphones of the speech-training amplifier, but gradually became interested in using sound-making toys near the microphone while the writer wore the headphones and he watched the decibel meter needle move. He then allowed the writer to talk and sing into the microphone while he listened.

Eventually, he did the 'go' test when wearing the headphones. At first he put a peg in when he heard the word and saw the decibel meter needle move, and later when listening alone with no visual clues. He would respond to 'go' even when it was unamplified if it reached him via the headphones, but still ignored it when he was not wearing them.

July and August (250–4,000 c/s 50–70 dB)

In another of Rees' games, L.S. was given four cards on which the following were drawn.

(1) An unbroken line   ————————————

(2) A broken line   — — — — —

(3) A dotted line   • • • • • • • • • •

(4) A zigzag line   ∧∧∧∧∧∧

L.S. was asked to show the card which associated with (1) a continuous note of 500 c/s (2) the same note given for one second at one second intervals (3) the note given in many short pips and (4) the note alternating each second with a higher note—1,000 c/s. L.S. quickly learned to do this.

September (250–4,000 c/s at 50–70 dB)

L.S. was now willing to wear headphones, and he was given a monaural pure tone test using the Ampilvox audiometer. He responded by saying in which ear the sound was 'in'. His response was much the same as in May.

	250	500	1k	2k	4k	c/s
Right ear	20	20	20	15	15	dB
Left ear	20	20	20	20	25	dB

October (250–4,000 c/s at 50–70 dB)

L.S. listened to the sound made by four toys—a drum, a clacker, a bell and a whistle, which covered the frequencies from 250–4,000 c/s. He turned his back, listened to one, turned around and said which it was. He recognized the sounds of another set of toys sounded at a quieter level (50–60 dB). Since he recognized them they were well above threshold.

The loud toys were used again the next day when L.S. was required to say which toy he heard without first playing with them to refresh his memory of the association of toy and sound. He recognized only the drum. After playing with them for a little while he again recognized them all.

November and December (250–4,000 c/s at 50–70 dB)

L.S. was beginning to use his voice quite playfully, imitating animal sounds, or the pitch of note, making sound as a signal to the writer to put a peg in a hole, pretending to telephone or talk, pretending to sing. He could now make quiet or loud vocal sounds.

January (250–4,000 c/s at 50–70 dB)

L.S. could now repeat a given sound sequence striking tin:box:cymbal or drum:drum:tin in the order shown. He willingly wore headphones while experimenting with sounds and was interested in making various vocal sounds into the microphone and hearing his own voice through the headphones. He enjoyed having a nursery rhythm record to put on the record player. He would march around the room with the other children marking the rhythm with cymbals, a triangle, whistle or a drum and changing his instrument from time to time. When he blew the whistle he would hum the note of it as he blew. When another boy was playing a 'three blind mice' rhythm on the melodica, L.S. began to hum to himself in time to the rhythm.

CASES QUOTED

February and March (250–4,000 c/s at 50–70 dB)

We felt that the time had come when we should begin to teach him to pay closer attention to sound. We therefore devised several special games for him.

L.S. had to listen carefully and show that he knew whether the sound was in the left ear or in the right ear. He was given a 'hundred counting tray' which had 10 rows and 10 spaces. He had a supply of counters, half of them green and the rest orange. He wore headphones which had green streamers attached to the right and orange streamers attached to the left. Working along the rows from left to right, he was required to put a green counter in when he heard a sound in his right ear—an orange counter when he heard it in the left. A small sweet was placed in the last space of the row upon which he was working.

(1) For a signal, a high frequency sound (4,000 c/s) at 60 dB was given at first. After 30 goes this was stopped.

(a) His response was random.

(b) When he had picked up the counter he looked at the writer for approval. If the writer did not approve immediately, he was quite ready to change it for the other colour, whether he was right or wrong.

(c) The writer did not know whether L.S. could not attend to the sound or whether he heard it but could not say in which ear the sound was in.

(2) The writer first made sure that L.S. could respond to 500 c/s at 60 dB and then used this for the signal. He showed unmistakably that he could hear this well.

(a) He sang the note spontaneously.

(b) He spontaneously imitated the duration of the sound.

———————— aaah!

— — — — — — ugh ugh ugh

•••••••••• u u u u u

145

The writer then established that L.S. was to make the decision as to which ear the sound was in without referring to the writer. To do this he had a small dish. If he responded to the sound the writer put a sweet in. The writer kept him waiting, and if he 'responded' when there was no sound, one sweet was taken out.

(3) We then returned to the left/right game using 500 c/s. In 30 goes he got most of them right with occasional errors. When he attended closely he could demonstrate that he knew whether a sound was in the left or right ear by using colour clues.

Although L.S. was now responding well to mechanical sounds, he was not attending to speech. A game was devised which showed clearly that he was 'cutting out' human voice. He was again given the 'hundred counting tray'. The score sheet was drawn out in 80 squares. Each square was marked with the sound which was to be given. Four different sounds were given in random order.

(1) Hammer loudly knocked under the table so that L.S. could both hear and feel it.

(2) Voice close to his ear so that he could both hear it and feel the breath.

(3) Quiet hammer tap under the writer's chair which L.S. could hear but not feel.

(4) Loud voice calling him by name.

The scores for (1) and (2) were not counted. He responded to these every time because an extra clue was given. (3) and (4) were done 30 times each and response to these was scored as follows.

quiet hammer	26 out of 30
loud voice	nil out of 30

He responded to all mechanical sounds but cut out the writer's voice each time. In order to make him attend to voice we played lively games in which mechanical sounds were interspersed with words. He had to put out a counter when he heard any sound, bells, knocks, speech sounds, animal sounds, his own name, and words such as 'put one' 'another one', or 'one more'. L.S. quickly understood and responded well.

April (250–4,000 c/s at 50–70 dB)

Another game required L.S. to attend closely to sound and to show that he could distinguish between high and low sounds. A red whistle (1,500 c/s at 70–80 dB) and a black handled freefield audiometer (250 c/s at 65 dB) were used. He learned to associate red counters with the whistle and black counters with the audiometer. Further to this the next day the whistle was discarded and he responded to high and low tones on the audiometer by putting out red and black counters. He showed that he could now attend to voice and distinguish between two words. He associated 'yes!' (with rising intonation) with the act of put a counter in and 'no!' (with falling intonation) with 'don't put one', at first watching for a nod or a shake of the head and then with the words said behind him.

Although L.S. was still understanding no spoken language, his general progress in the classroom was good. He was beginning to recognize printed words and to copy them. His drawing and handwork and play were good. He was beginning to imitate words and to attempt to use them. He was very happy and lively and a good placement was found for him.

These cases have been selected to show as wide a variety as possible of the many problems encountered in assessing the hearing of disturbed children. Each case is unique and the investigation must take a different line with each child towards finding the way to make him demonstrate what he hears.

11—Classroom Work at the Belmont Hospital Children's Units

Joan E. Taylor

PRACTICAL GAMES

The work in the classroom is experimental in approach and the teaching programme is continually being adapted to suit each different child. Since the children do not comprehend spoken language the simple tasks must be presented in such a way that they explain themselves to a child without the help of verbal instruction.

The games here described are mainly concerned with concepts of colour, shape and size. Most of the children readily occupy themselves with things they can handle, and will make primitive arrangements of these, piling them up or setting them in a line, and this offered a line of approach. Few children fail to observe, imitate and continue in making simple order of different kinds when this is demonstrated to them. They are able to pile up, put on, take off, put in, take out, put red on red and blue on blue, put square here and round there; to match, sort, fit and arrange two or three dimensional coloured shapes. Even at this early stage some of the handicapping difficulties are already apparent. These include the perceptual difficulty of a child who cannot orient shapes, the clumsy, fumbling handling of material by the dyspraxic child, the inability of the distractible child, highly sensitive to all perceptual input to direct and focus his attention on what is relevant. The most common difficulty, however, is inattention to the matter in hand.

The demands of the classroom are different from the demands of daily life. The daily routine which is the same each day and the simple social habits and skills with cup, spoon and toothbrush are matters of association memory and habit formation. But in the classroom different demands are made each day. Various challenging situations require alertness and observation from the child, and require that he should adjust to different situations, now attend to colours, now to shapes; see differences or similarities, make order in this way or in that, recall things shown and hidden and respond to many such demands. The child is required to pay attention. These are some of the difficulties the children exhibit which prevent them from giving more than cursory attention to data offered.

(1) Some children use the activities to 'cut out' the teacher. They work hard, but because they will not accept suggestions, they repeat over and over again the same simple play. It takes patience to intrude gradually until the child accepts the teacher's interference and rapport is established.

(2) There is the deliberate inattention of the child who attempts to use the situation to manipulate the behaviour of the teacher.

(3) There is often a partial withdrawal from a situation showing apparent reluctance to get involved in a situation which requires mental effort.

(4) There may be a rigidity or 'stickiness' of mind which causes a child to remember too well what he has just done instead of giving fresh attention to the next item. This probably shows that the child is unable to analyse a complex command such as 'choose a square and put it on the square' into its two demands of 'choose and put' combined with 'square' and so he repeats the whole action instead of seeing that the next demand is 'choose and put' combined with 'round'.

(5) Many of the children have difficulty in scanning the material offered and choosing the significant item; for example, when pairing identical objects, 'find another one like this one', a child may pick up every wrong one and ignore the right as though, because he is holding in his mind an image of what he is looking for, he cannot see that it is 'also' on the table. By patiently giving a child the time he requires to consider the simple problem and encouraging him to persist until he has finished it, one can help him to enjoy co-operating in a series of simple games.

Remembering colour or shape

If one wants to know whether a child remembers a colour it is necessary to give him a choice of being right or wrong, so in the game here described two colours are used. Two identical open-ended boxes are placed before the child. One face of one is brown, one face of the other is yellow. Two dozen two inch square cards are used, half of them brown and half yellow.

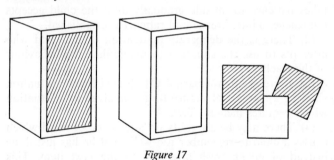

Figure 17

There are three steps in the game.

(1) The coloured side of the boxes faces the child. He is handed the coloured squares one at a time in random order and posts them into the appropriate box until he gets three or four right.

150

(2) The boxes are then turned round with the coloured side facing away from the child but in the same position as regards left and right. The child has now to remember the colours of the boxes as he continues to post the squares. If he succeeds in this he attempts the next step.

(3) Without looking again at the colours on the boxes the child watches them being switched over to change places. He continues to post the cards into the boxes in their new positions. Some children remember when the box is first turned round but have difficulty in continuing to remember. Similar games can be played with different shapes.

APPLICATION OF VISUAL MEMORY

(1) Various games are used to find out whether the children can apply visual memory in doing a more difficult task. In the third step of the game just described the children are required to remember the colours and to 'switch' them mentally.

(2) In this next game the child must link his visual memory of an object with a memory of what the object feels like. A curtained, wooden box is placed before the child. Pairs of little solid shapes are used. One of each shape is given to the child who examines it, looks at it and feels it and puts it in the box.

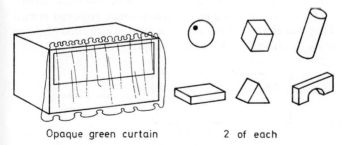

Opaque green curtain   2 of each

Figure 18

When one of each shape is in the box, the child is shown one shape which is placed on top of the box. He feels in the box for the matching shape. Some children have considerable difficulty. They confuse not only the right angled objects but the concave surface of the 'bridge' with the convex surface of the ball and cylinder.

(3) Another game in this group presents the child with four objects, each of distinctive shape and different colour. When he has examined them and put them into the curtained box he is shown a coloured card. He must remember which object was that colour and find it by feeling in the box.

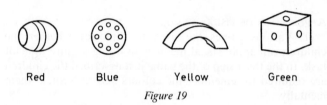

| Red | Blue | Yellow | Green |

Figure 19

DEALING WITH TWO CONCEPTS

Many of the children have difficulty in dealing with two concepts at once. Even this next game, which is essentially only a matching game, some of the children found difficult because it required them to deal with both colour and shape.

(1) The children are given various small, coloured bricks. They are shown cards, one at a time, which 'describe' the brick by stating its colour and shape.

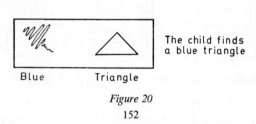

The child finds a blue triangle

Blue   Triangle

Figure 20

152

Several of the children matched the shape, and then matched the colour a number of times before finding one which satisfied both, and they continued to do this with each new card.

(2) Here is another game which many of the children have found difficult. They are given a tray of little coloured rods. Cards are presented one at a time. Each card has two small coloured circles drawn on it. The child stands a rod on each circle, matching the colour.

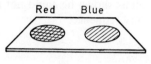

Figure 21

Several of the children perceived one of the colours (for example, red) saw that there were two circles, so took two red rods, put one on, saw that the other did not match, so exchanged it for a blue one, and continued to work in this way for each card.

This difficulty in dealing efficiently with two concepts at one time even in simple matching games, shows in many other games which deal with shape and colour, shape and size, colour and size, although the children can deal with colour, shape or size by itself. The difficulty increases in games which require the child to recall one concept while the other is present.

SERIATION BY SIZE

Various games are given which require the child to put things in order of size, building towers and steps, arranging cards, sticks, buttons, shells, stones and shapes. A 'model' of the concept is given to help the child to place things in diminishing order, and this can be turned round.

SEQUENCING MEMORY

Another group of games in this series requires the child to show that he can reconstruct sequences of two or three items which are presented and then taken away. There seem to be several reasons why the children find this difficult. Some cannot pay sufficient attention, others remember too well the first sequence shown and cannot forget it when presented with another sequence. One boy could remember several sequences if they were given silently, but if the items were named as well as shown he could not remember more than one item in any sequence.

REPEATING A PATTERN

A group of games which the children find very difficult is that which requires them to deal with repeating a pattern, first by building many units of the pattern and then putting these in sequence; and also by breaking down given patterns into units. Even after many different exercises the children do not make any generalization which would enable them to tackle a new pattern by themselves. All their old difficulties re-appear. One of the simplest repeating patterns is alternating the following pattern.

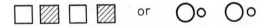

Figure 22

Many of the children do not see this as a unit repeated, but try to match the last item with another similar one. The exercise demands that the child should deal with 'twoness', two different colours, and with left and right and all this is confused by the concepts of repetition.

A pattern of 'one orange square two blue square' embodies choice of colour, choice of number, spatial position, the concept of three items being part of a whole, and the concept of repetition of the unit. Even if a child learned 'by heart' to repeat a pattern of 'one orange square two squares blue,' if the same basic pattern is given with either shapes or colours changed it is a wholly new problem to the child. He does not generalize. This exercise gave the child so much difficulty that some very simple games were given to try to find out why they found it so hard.

A card with a pattern of red alternating circles and squares drawn on it was given to a child, together with a box of round and square beads.

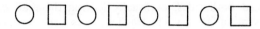

Figure 23

(1) The child could not start at the first and work one by one along to the end.

(2) He would keep closing up the row, pushing the beads along until they touched each other.

(3) If he had just put a round one—even while pointing to the next square—he would take another round one.

Most of the children did these things, and not once but continually.

To help the children further other little games were devised—a number of 1 inch card squares were made—half of them purple and the rest green. On the back of the purple ones there was a red ring; on the back of the green there was a green cross. Starting at the left we made a long row alternating purple and green. The child was then asked to turn over every purple one—showing the red things. He then turned over every green one. He then substituted a red counter for every purple one and so we kept going over the line—altering the pattern.

SUBSTITUTION

A simple game of substitution gave the children much less trouble. It involves visual memory and visual association. Twenty-four cards 1½ inches square were prepared—8 red, 8 black and 8 yellow with symbols drawn on the back.

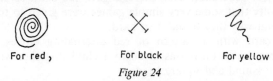

For red,   For black   For yellow

Figure 24

Four of each colour were given to the child and he examined both sides, eventually leaving them all on the table, symbol face up. The teacher places a red card, colour side up and asked the child to find one of his red ones. He finds the spiral, turns it over and puts it by the teacher's card.

ANALOGIES

Analogies is a game played with some of the children's bricks. Green and red bricks are used. Some 1½ inch cards are prepared—one is red and one is green, and for each shape an outline is drawn on one card and a blacked-in outline on another. The game is played on an 8 inch square divided into 4. Two bricks and one card are placed and the child finds the fourth.

An extension of the analogies game is the building of simple matrices, placing pattern against colour, toy against colour, and so on. Several suggestions for cue matching games were made by Rees, notably a series of games dealing with cues for concept, the most popular of which was 'red for hot', 'blue for cold'.

(1) Two large glass jars were filled with water, one hot, one cold. Red powder paint was dropped into the hot one.

The child held the jar and watched it mix. Blue was put into the cold similarly.

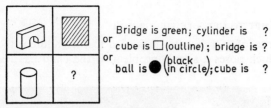

Bridge is green; cylinder is   ?
or   cube is ☐ (outline) ; bridge is ?
or   ball is ● (black in circle); cube is   ?

Figure 25

(2) Two small identical bottles, one red, filled with hot, one blue filled with cold, were put in the curtained box. When the child was shown a red card he felt in the box for the hot one.

(3) Ten small identical bottles filled with clear water, five hot and five cold were given to the child. He felt each bottle and put collars on them, red for hot and blue for cold.

(4) We went round the house looking for hot and cold things and the child said whether they were red or blue.

BIG AND SMALL SYMBOLS

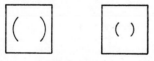

Figure 26

Big and small symbols were associated with a hand sign for the big one and finger sign for the small one. Some of the children could choose a larger or smaller toy when shown the card or when shown the hand or finger sign. A few children when shown one of two objects could 'say' it was small or large by using finger sign or hand sign, but

157

when a bottle or brick or button which had been small became 'big' by being associated with a smaller one, the children were confused.

ATTEMPT TO GET 'OFF THE GROUND'

Series of exercises are presented to the children, the last of which poses a simple problem. If the child has learned

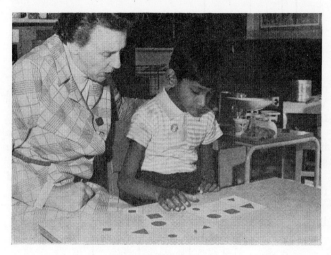

Figure 27. Teaching games.

anything from the exercises and can analyse and apply what he has learned he should be able to solve the problem. The simplest of these consists of a number of card strips on each of which is drawn a simple repeat pattern of coloured squares and circles on which the child places cut out coloured squares and discs. On the last few cards the final items are not coloured and the child must judge how to complete the row.

The main purpose of all these games is to give the children some sense of order and structure and practice in dealing with things in an orderly way. Commonly these children show lack of drive, lack of curiosity and too much dependence on adults to structure their learning. If games can be devised which lead the child on to a point where he

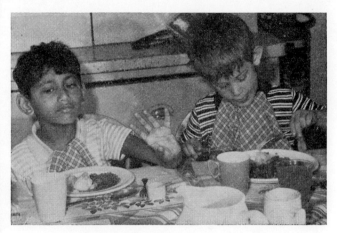

Figure 28. Negative and positive attitudes to food.

himself can discover the final solution, it might spark off in him learning of a quality which cannot be taught by rote learning or learning at second hand. However carefully a series of games is planned, each time we arrive at a point where it seems the child must take off—he doesn't. But there is some increased awareness and adaptability. The children become better able to cope and begin to communicate.

It seems that all the bits of information we acquire do not cohere or coalesce into a structured whole unless there is a live nucleus of original thought. Word labelling is not language. Word recognition is not reading. Articulation of speech is not talking. Working through these little structured games is not problem solving. A chimp can do the first in each case, but only man the second. The first is a matter of association memory, the second is activity of a wholly different order.

12—Research

Dr. Ian Evans, Ph.D.

CURRENT TECHNIQUES

In 1966 the Nuffield Provincial Hospitals' Trust awarded a
research grant to Dr. Louis Minski to study the possibilities
of teaching autistic children using principles of learning and
perception derived from experimental psychology. A number
of experimental case reports in the literature suggested that
the formal, systematic application of operant conditioning
principles, or behaviour modification techniques, was
effective in eliminating particular behaviour problems in
severely disturbed children and in building up simple
patterns of behaviour. The clinical research on this topic
has since grown considerably, and after reviewing the
literature Leff (1968) concluded the following.

> The results of these studies indicate that behavior-modifica-
> tion techniques may be extremely useful tools in the education
> and rehabilitation of psychotic children. None of the investi-
> gators whose work was reviewed here would claim that they
> have cured their subjects. But many can justifiably state that
> they have equipped their subjects with several of the basic
> skills and habits necessary for the most rudimentary of
> adjustments to their social environment. Furthermore,
> behavior 'therapists', guided by social-learning models which
> are more parsimonious than traditional psychodynamic
> theories, have been able to effectively control, and in several

cases eliminate, much of the undesirable and maladaptive behavior of these children. Results such as these, achieved with types of patients that had formerly proven largely intractable to other therapeutic approaches, are sufficient to warrant further exploratory research in this area.

Thus behaviour modification techniques seemed to offer a rational and easily definable method of treatment, and the Children's Unit offered an ideal, humane environment for the objective assessment of the efficacy of the method. It was decided to concentrate specifically on speech and language development for a number of reasons. Firstly, the children's speech could be objectively recorded for assessing the amount of progress achieved. Secondly, speech was unlikely, from past clinical observations, to develop spontaneously in the five year old autistic children concerned. Thirdly, evidence was accumulating that the language deficit was *the* deficit, or one of the primary, deficits of psychotic children (Rutter, 1968); fourthly, most important, of the children concerned none had any communicative speech.

Three autistic children with average intellectual potential on non-verbal testing were selected for the first stage of this research, which was carried out by the Research Psychologist, Dr. J. Humphery, and supervised by Dr. H. N. M. Rees, Consultant Child Psychiatrist. The diagnostic label of the autistic syndrome of early childhood was applied independently by the two consultant psychiatrists. The clinical status of the children was described in detail (Rees and colleagues, 1968) their intellectual potential tested in depth by the educational psychologist, and their general social behaviour documented by a rating scale filled out for each child by all the members of staff. Before therapy began one child had no meaningful words, one had some twenty words recognizable only to the parents, and the third had a a few very distorted dyslalic sounds which he had acquired slowly from the age of eighteen months. Improvement was

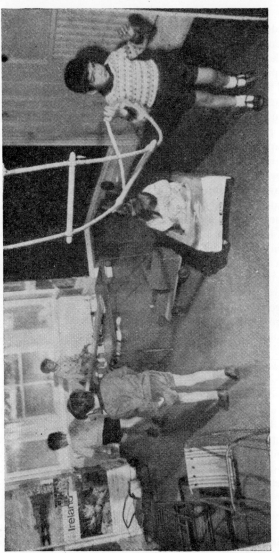

Figure 29. The playroom in one of the units.

recorded by word-counts during the tape-recorded therapy sessions, a check-list of words or sounds was made outside the therapy room, and the regular reports of the speech therapist were studied.

All three children were severely disturbed and difficult to manage. Their visual avoidance was so severe that at the start of the therapy it was necessary to shape even the most basic response of observing visual stimuli. This was done by using the simple repetitive rocking habits of the children to manipulate a lever on a spring. Backwards and forwards pushes of this lever lit up in sequence a row of yellow lights—the row ended in a green light and when this was reached a bell sounded and a small chocolate sweet dropped into a tray near the child's hand. A control panel for the therapist made it possible only to dispense a sweet contingent upon the child observing each light as it appeared.

Once this had been achieved the speech therapy began with the child's attention now being directed towards coloured photographic slides projected in front of him on a large screen in a darkened room. The child sat inside a hardboard booth to reduce the possibly chaotic visual environment to the therapist's face and the large bright slides. The children sat on small comfortable chairs. One, who was extremely hyperactive, was restrained gently in a baby's high-chair. The slides were all photographs of common objects from the home—staff members, other children, parts of the body, items of food, clothing, and toys. They were bright and clear against suitable neutral backgrounds. The spoken names of the objects were presented to the child by means of a tape recorder synchronized with the slides. The children wore for this purpose soft earphones which brought the stimulus as close as possible and also cut out other distracting background noises. The slides and tape combination did tend to elicit from the child whatever sounds were in their limited repertoires. Initially, any sound made was immediately

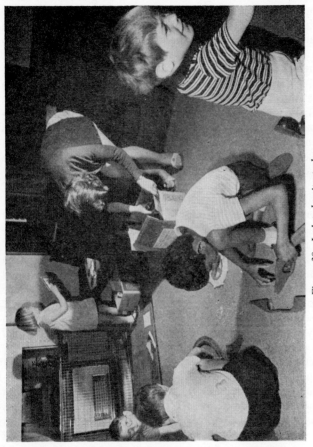

Figure 30. Isolated unit at play.

165

reinforced with a small piece of chocolate or other food that the children liked. Then a shaping procedure was employed, that is, the systematic rewarding of sounds which approximate the desired word. Sessions lasted about 40 minutes with a ten-minute break in between. After a mean number of 50 sessions (about a six-month period as only two sessions per week were given) all three children were rated as improved by the staff. One child acquired a meaningful vocabulary of over 300 words which generalized well to the home situation. There was considerable spontaneity in his speech and he could produce novel phrases and combinations of words which were used appropriately. His Vineland age increased by 15 months and the child was discharged to a residential school for children with language disorders. The second child also showed a Vineland increase of 15 months, but his words were only 'word labellings' and dyslalic—although he made differentiated sounds they were not comprehensible. Similarly, the third child would respond with a differentiated sound to each slide but few of them could be considered acceptable words.

These two children then had a second series of speech training sessions in which the earphones were dispensed with and an attempt was made to teach the children a basic repertoire of English speech sounds. At this stage the new research psychologist, Ian M. Evans and a visiting American psychologist, Rosemary Nelson, incorporated traditional speech therapy techniques and designed a set of visual/ tactile cues which aided the child in producing the correct sound and also aided him in the discrimination of one speech-sound from another. Once the speech-sounds had been acquired it was possible to sequence them into words. This was still done with the coloured slides and the reinforcement of sweets. After 20 more sessions one child had mastered the complete set of speech-sounds and after a further 25 sessions he had a vocabulary of well over 200 words which generalized to both the unit and the child's own home.

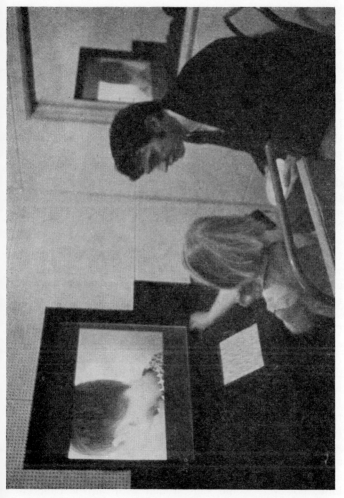

Figure 31. Operant conditioning.

167

Improvement was shown in both complexity and spontaneity of speech on the two relevant items on the rating scale.

The other child, however, although he learned each speech-sound, could not sequence them into words and could not learn to pair any particular sound consistently with an object. At the same time his previous dyslalic utterances greatly reduced as they were no longer reinforced. Attempts were made briefly to increase motivational level by using his lunch as a reinforcer, but after a total of 26 sessions the therapy was abandoned. One reason for this was that the parallel assessment and information from staff and teachers demonstrated that the child still had severe perceptual difficulties and invariably failed any task involving more than one sense modality. It seemed irrational to persist in speech training when there were defects in processes basic to speech acquisition, and training procedures of a less ambitious kind were introduced, using simple perceptual tasks gradually increasing in complexity. Another reason was that the repeated failure seemed to be having an adverse effect on the child. We have noticed that psychotic children react emotionally to the experience of failure and there is some experimental evidence for this. Birch and Walker (1966) have shown the perceptual disintegration of psychotic children following failure on a task. In a Ph.D. thesis, Acker (1966) reports that autistic children can be taught discriminations in an errorless procedure that they could not be taught in the normal trial-and-error presentation. In errorless discrimination the negative stimulus is gradually faded in so that the organism continues to respond to the positive stimulus without ever making an error. One of the great advantages of operant principles is that the task is always broken down into small steps to ensure the minimum amount of error on the part of the subjects. Evidence of this kind, however, would suggest that with autistic children even more particular care has to be taken to ensure that the steps are broken down into suitable units. From this information alone the failure of traditional teaching methods is predictable.

The use of speech cues was tried in two other cases. One was a mute child with a language disorder (executive aphasia) complicated by a super-imposed elective mutism. He could make only two undifferentiated sounds, but by the end of the 15th session had acquired the complete repertoire. By the 29th session, when therapy had to be terminated, he had about 20 clear words, used appropriately, but the volume of these was well below normal. Another child with executive aphasia and an educationally subnormal level of intelligence, had a large vocabulary of words and the speech cues were used to improve his articulation. After 21 sessions his articulation had improved considerably, he was able to correct himself if negative feedback followed a poorly articulated word, and the staff rated both the complexity and spontaneity of speech as improved (Nelson and Evans, 1968).

Since then most of the work has been concentrated on using the technology of operant learning to set up a controlled testing situation for a more reliable and valid assessment of the child's learning and/or perceptual difficulties than is at present possible with the standardized psychological tests. The laboratory consists of three rooms, converted from two spare bedrooms in one of the houses of the unit. One room is the therapy room, semi-soundproofed and equipped with acoustic tiles. It contains a large back-projection screen above the testing console. Alongside this room is the observation room with a one-way mirror and intercom facilities to listen to the children or to communicate with the therapist. The control room contains the slide projector, tape recorders, cumulative recorder for measuring the children's responses, Smartie dispensers for delivering sweets into the therapy room, and the key element, the programming equipment. This is a versatile logical module

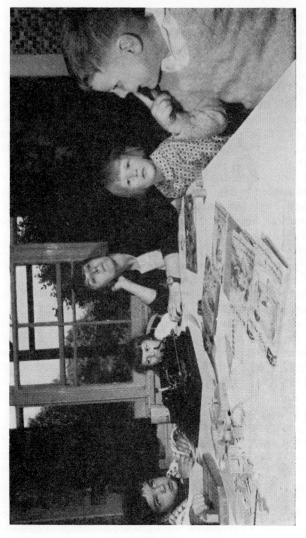

Figure 32. Helping to develop speech continues throughout the day.

system of the type commonly found in experimental psychology laboratories. It allows integration between the various interchangeable manipulanda mounted on the console (such as levers and push-buttons) the various stimuli possible (such as coloured lights, picture slides, match-to-sample problems, tones, words, music or virtually any kind of complex stimuli required) and the reinforcements—sweets, tokens, new problems, door-chimes and so on (Evans, 1969).

This equipment provides an environment for the speech and language development that is easy to regulate and which has already proved extremely valuable. It remains to be seen whether it can usefully provide automatic testing facilities for understanding the complex perceptual and cognitive difficulties underlying the severe language disorders revealed by the children.

Appendix

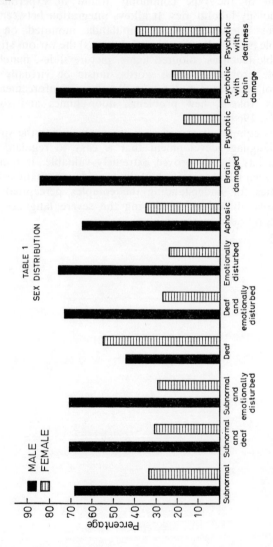

TABLE 1
SEX DISTRIBUTION

TABLE 2
FAMILY HISTORY (PERCENTAGES)

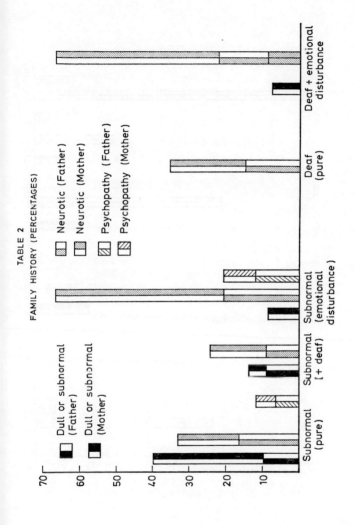

Legend:
- Neurotic (Father)
- Neurotic (Mother)
- Psychopathy (Father)
- Psychopathy (Mother)
- Dull or subnormal (Father)
- Dull or subnormal (Mother)

Categories (x-axis):
- Subnormal (pure)
- Subnormal (+ deaf)
- Subnormal (emotional disturbance)
- Deaf (pure)
- Deaf + emotional disturbance

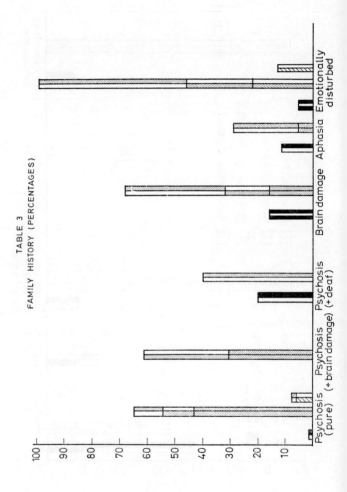

TABLE 3
FAMILY HISTORY (PERCENTAGES)

174

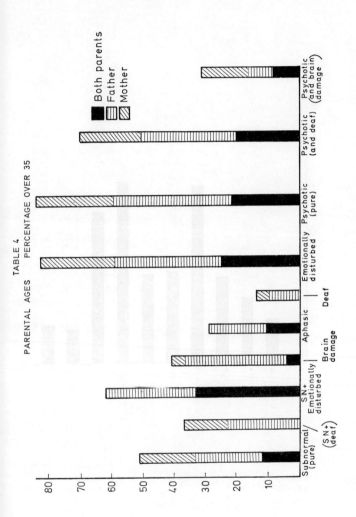

TABLE 4

PARENTAL AGES   PERCENTAGE OVER 35

Both parents
Father
Mother

Subnormal/(pure) (S N+ deaf) | Emotionally disturbed S N+ | Brain damage | Aphasic | Deaf | Emotionally disturbed | Psychotic (pure) | Psychotic (and deaf) | Psychotic (and brain damage)

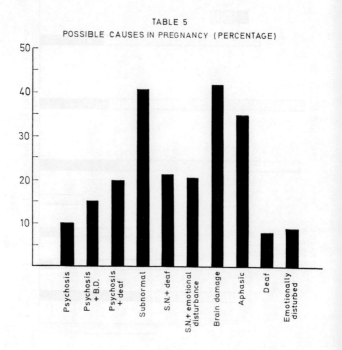

TABLE 5
POSSIBLE CAUSES IN PREGNANCY (PERCENTAGE)

TABLE 6

POSSIBLE PERINATAL CAUSES (PERCENTAGE)

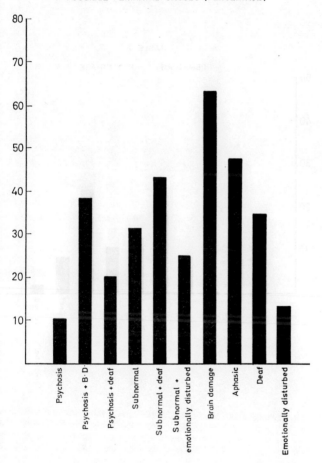

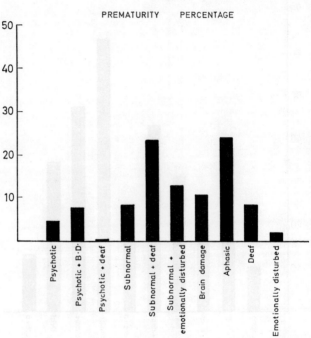

TABLE 7

PREMATURITY   PERCENTAGE

TABLE 8

POSSIBLE CAUSATIVE INTERCURRENT ILLNESS (PERCENTAGE)

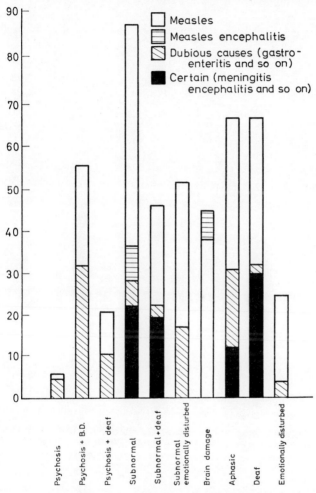

REFERENCES

Acker, L. E. (1966). Errorless Discrimination Training in Autistic and Normal Children, *Dissertation Abstracts*, **27** (6–B) 2152.

Annell, A. L. (1963). The Prognosis of Psychotic Syndromes in Children, *Acta. psychiat. Scand.*, **39**, 235.

Barber, D. S. P. and Edwards, J. H. (1967). *Br. med. J.*, **38,** 695.

Bartlett, F. C. (1932). London; Cambridge University Press.

Birch, H. G. and Walker, H. A. (1966). *Archs gen. Psychiat.*, **14,** 113–118.

Bowlby, J. (1951). Families of Psychotic Children. *J. Child Psychol. Psychiat.*, **1,** 56.

Creak, M. (1961). The Schizophrenic Syndrome in Childhood, *Br. med. J.*, **2,** 889–890.

—— and Ini, S. (1960). Families of Psychotic Children. *J. Child Psychol. Psychiat.*, **1,** 56.

—— and working party (1961). *Schizophrenic Syndrome in Childhood.* Progress report.

Eisenberg, L. and Kanner, L. (1956). *Am. J. Orthopsychiat.*, **26,** 556–66.

Evans, I. M. (1969). *A Modular Teaching Unit for Research and Therapy with Children.* Unpublished report; Belmont Hospital Children's Units.

Goldfarb, W. (1964). *Arch gen. Psychiat.*, **11,** 620–34.

Hanley, W. (1968). Unpublished report addressed to the Society for Paediatric Research, Atlantic City, New Jersey.

Henderson, P. (1968). *Milroy Lectures.*

Luria, A. R. and Vinogradova, O. S. (1959). The Dynamics of Semantic Systems, *Br. J. Psychol.*, **50,** 89.

Leff, R. (1968). *Psychological Bulletin*, **69**, 396–409.

REFERENCES

Lennette, E. H. (1968). Unpublished report addressed to the Annual General Meeting of American Societies for Experimental Biology, Atlantic City, New Jersey.

Maucaulay, D. and Watson, M. (1967). *Archs Dis. Childh.*, **42**, 225.

Mauser, H. M., Wolff, J. A., Firster, M., Poppers, P. S., Rantuck, E., Kuntzmann, R. and Connery, A. H. (1968). *Lancet*, **2**, 122.

National Society for Mentally Handicapped Children (1967). *Stress in Families with a Mentally Handicapped Child*, Report, London; The National Society for Mentally Handicapped Children.

Nelson, R. O. and Evans, I. M. (1968). *J. Child Psychol. Psychiat.*, **9**, 111–124.

O'Gorman, G. (1967). *The Nature of Childhood Autism*, London; Butterworths; New York, Appleton-Century-Crofts, Inc.

Rees, H. N. M., Minski, L., Humphery, J., Bowley, A. H. and Evans, I. M. (1968). *Autism in Early Childhood—an Approach Towards a Rational Investigation and Therapeutic Care.* Unpublished report, Belmont Hospital Children's Units.

Rimland, B. (1964). *Infantile Autism.* New York; Appleton-Century-Crofts, Inc.

Rutter, M. (1968). *J. Child Psychol. Psychiat.*, **9**, 111–124.

Stephenson, J. P. B. and McBean, M. (1967). *Br. med. J.*, **3**, 579–581.

Tizard, J. (1964). *Community Services for the Mentally Handicapped.* London; Oxford University Press.

—— and Grad, J. C. (1961). *The Mentally Handicapped and their Families.* London; Oxford University Press.

Williams, M. (1968). *Brit. J. Disorders of Communication*, **3**, (1) 60.

Wing, J. K. (1966). *Early Childhood Autism; Clinical, Educational and Social Aspects.* London; Pergamon Press.

Index